HEALING YOUR GRIEVING BODY

Also by Alan Wolfelt:

Creating Meaningful Funeral Ceremonies: A Guide for Families

Healing a Child's Grieving Heart: 100 Practical Ideas for Families, Friends and Caregivers

Healing a Friend's Grieving Heart: 100 Practical Ideas for Helping Someone You Love Through Loss

Healing Your Grieving Heart for Kids: 100 Practical Ideas

The Journey Through Grief: Reflections on Healing

Understanding Your Grief: Ten Essential Touchstones for Finding Hope and Healing Your Heart

The Wilderness of Grief: Finding Your Way

Companion Press is dedicated to the education and support of both the bereaved and bereavement caregivers. We believe that those who companion the bereaved by walking with them as they journey in grief have a wondrous opportunity: to help others embrace and grow through grief—and to lead fuller, more deeply-lived lives themselves because of this important ministry.

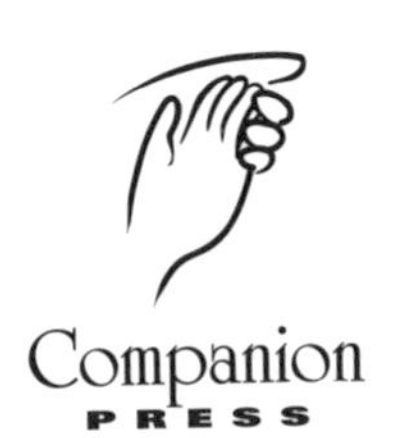

For a complete catalog and ordering information, write or call:

Companion Press
The Center for Loss and Life Transition
3735 Broken Bow Road
Fort Collins, CO 80526
(970) 226-6050
www.centerforloss.com

HEALING YOUR GRIEVING BODY

•

100 PHYSICAL PRACTICES FOR MOURNERS

Simple mind-body activities to help you care for yourself when you are grieving

•

ALAN D. WOLFELT, PH.D.

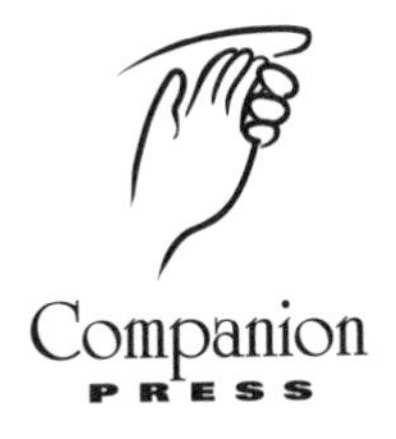

Companion
PRESS

Fort Collins, Colorado

An imprint of the Center for Loss and Life Transition

Companion Press is an imprint of the
Center for Loss and Life Transition,
3735 Broken Bow Road, Fort Collins, Colorado 80526
970-226-6050
www.centerforloss.com

Companion Press books may be purchased in bulk for sales promotions, premiums or fundraisers. Please contact the publisher at the above address for more information.

Printed in the United States of America

12 11 10 09 5 4 3 2 1

ISBN: 978-1-879651-63-0

INTRODUCTION

"And no one ever told me about the laziness of grief."
– C.S. Lewis

This book is in your hands because you are in mourning. You have been "torn apart" and have some very special needs right now. Among these special needs is to nurture yourself in five important ways: physically; emotionally; cognitively; socially; and spiritually. While all of these areas are vitally important, this book focuses on practical ways to nurture yourself in the physical realm.

When you are in mourning, you usually feel under-rested and overwhelmed. Your body is probably letting you know it feels distress. You may feel you have no strength left for your own basic needs, let alone the needs of others. Actually, one literal definition of the word "grievous" is "causing physical suffering." Yes, right now your body is telling you it has, just like your heart, been torn apart and has some special needs!

Your body is so very wise. It will try to slow you down and invite you to authentically mourn the losses that touch your life. The emotions of grief are often experienced as bodily-felt energies. We mourn life losses from the inside out. In our experience as a physician and grief counselor, it is only when we care for ourselves physically that we can integrate our losses emotionally and spiritually. Allow us to introduce you to how your body attempts to slow you down and prepare you to mourn your life losses.

Among the most common physical responses to loss are trouble sleeping and low energy. It is so common we even have a fancy term for it—the "lethargy of grief." You are probably finding that your normal sleep patterns have been thrown off. Perhaps you are having difficulty getting to sleep, but even more commonly, you may wake up early in the morning and have trouble getting back to sleep. During your grief journey your body needs more rest than usual. You may also find yourself getting tired more quickly—sometimes even at the start of the day.

Sleeping normally after a loss would be unusual. If you think about it, sleep is the primary way in which we release control. When you experience a life loss, you feel a great loss of control. At a subconscious level, you may not want to lose any more control by sleeping. So sleep problems are very natural in the face of life losses.

Muscle aches and pains, shortness of breath, feelings of emptiness in your stomach, tightness in your throat or chest, digestive problems, sensitivity to noise, heart palpitations, queasiness, nausea, headaches, increased allergy symptoms, changes in appetite, weight loss or gain, agitation, and generalized tension—these are all ways your body may react to losses that you encounter in life.

The stress of grief can suppress your immune system and make you more vulnerable to physical problems. If you have a chronic existing health challenge, it may become worse. Right now you may not feel in control of how your body is responding. Your body is communicating with you about the special needs it has right now. Befriending and mindfully giving attention to your physical symptoms will allow you to discover your body's native intelligence.

Yet, it can be difficult to slow down and care for your body when you are surrounded by common societal messages that tell us to be strong in the face of grief. Have you had anyone tell you things like, "Keep busy," "Carry on," or "You need to put the past in the past"? These and other similar messages often discourage you from practicing physical self-care, which, by contrast, is needed because it invites you to suspend. In actuality, when you are in mourning, you need to slow down, to turn inward, to embrace feelings of loss, and to seek and accept support. No, it is not always easy to care for your physical being in a mourning-avoidant culture. Without doubt, physical self-care takes time, mindfulness, and discernment.

You must realize that physical self-care is vitally important to you right now or you probably would not have picked up this book. As you know, your body is the house you live in. Just as your house requires care and maintenance to protect you from outside elements, your body requires that you honor it and be kind and gentle to it. The quality of your life ahead depends on how you care for your body today. The lethargy of grief you are probably experiencing is a natural mechanism intended to slow you down and encourage you to care for your body.

To practice physical self-care doesn't mean you are feeling sorry for yourself; rather it means you are allowing yourself to have the courage to pay attention to your special needs. For it is in physically nurturing yourself that you can eventually allow yourself the time and loving attention you need to journey through your grief to discover a fullness of living and loving again. That is why we encourage anyone who is in the midst of grief to put "nurture my physical self" right at the top of the daily to-do list.

Taking care of your physical self during this naturally vulnerable time in your life is essentially about personal guardianship. It means accepting personal responsibility for your own special health needs as part of your need to self-nurture. We are honored to provide you some information that we believe can and will help you in this endeavor, but just as your body is yours, so is the responsibility you have to care for it.

Right now your "divine spark"—that which gives your life meaning and purpose—may feel like it has been muted or even turned completely off. In large part, our hope is that this book helps your "physical switch" stay on, even if part of you wants to keep it in the off position. You see, we believe if we can help you take care of your physical body, over time and with no rewards for speed, your spirit, your "life force" or divine spark, can be re-ignited, and you can find renewed meaning and even joy in your life.

So, self-care is about being reminded to care for your body with the right actions, right living, and right thinking. You will practice self-care when you believe that you deserve it and when you love yourself enough to carry it out. The presence of daily, thoughtful care of your grieving body is a clear reflection of your holiness, and a lack of self-care represents an internal disregard for your being. So, as difficult as it may be for you right now, caring for your body is vital to your temporary surviving and your longer-term thriving.

How To Use This Book

As promised, this book contains 100 physical practices to soothe your body, calm your mind, and tend to your heart. Of course, caring for our physical bodies can be somewhat different for each of us. So, if you come to an idea that doesn't fit you, ignore it and flip to another page. However, you may want to stay open to trying some new physical self-care practices and see what happens.

You'll also notice that each of the 100 ideas offers a "carpe diem," which means "seize the day." Our hope is that you will not relegate this book to a shelf, but instead keep it handy on your nightstand or coffee table. Pick it up often and turn to any page; the carpe diem might help you seize the day by giving you a physical practice, action, or insight to consider today, right now, right this minute.

We hope that the 100 physical practices and principles in this resource encourage you to nurture yourself in ways that bring hope and healing.

1.

FOCUS ON SIMPLE SURVIVAL

- After the loss of someone you care about, you often feel shock, a psychic numbing of your senses, and a physical slowing of your body. You are taken down to your very basic needs of physical, emotional, and spiritual survival. Even the simplest acts of your life seem harder.
- Your body is wise in this natural slowing down. Well-intentioned people may try to divert you from this turning inward. Society often seems to have the expectation that we take off a day or two for a funeral, and then we immediately go back to work and "keep busy."
- But your body is giving you the opposite message: to turn inward and suspend activity for a period of time. Physically you must focus on your simple survival needs. Breathe in, breathe out, rest, provide your body with nourishment, drink fluids, and focus on what you need to get through this day.

CARPE DIEM:

Take the time to take a deep breath in and out. What do you need to get through this day? Are you getting enough food, water, and rest to keep your body healthy?

2.

MAKE AN INVENTORY OF SURVIVAL STRATEGIES

- What has helped you cope with stress and loss in the past? These strategies will probably help now, too.
- Make a list of the most difficult times in your life and the ways in which you helped yourself live through them. Did you spend time with family? Turn to your faith? Help take care of someone else? How did you take care of your body? Can you make use of any of these survival techniques today?
- Knowing what calms you is also important. Getting a massage, taking a walk, going for a swim, talking to your sister on the phone, walking the dog, meditating—find what works for you.

CARPE DIEM:

Make a list of what you need to get through the next month. Ask your friends and family to help you meet these needs.

3.

ALLOW FOR NUMBNESS

- Feelings of shock, numbness, and disbelief are nature's way of temporarily protecting us from the full reality of the death of someone loved. Like anesthesia, they help us survive the pain of our early grief. Be thankful for numbness.

- We often think, "I will wake up and this will not have happened." Early mourning can feel like being in a dream. Your emotions will need time to catch up with what your mind has been told. Your body, too, slows down in response to this emotional shock.

- Feelings of passivity often go hand-in-hand with numbness. You may feel child-like and need to be fed, dressed, and led through the day. You may neglect the most basic needs of your body, like food and water. You may even need others to make simple decisions for you.

- Even after you have moved beyond these initial feelings, don't be surprised if they reemerge. Birthdays, holidays, and anniversaries often trigger these normal and necessary feelings. Or sometimes, feelings of shock and numbness will surface for no apparent reason.

CARPE DIEM:

If you are feeling numb, cancel any commitments that require concentration and decision-making. Allow yourself time to regroup. Find a "safe haven" that you might be able to retreat to for a few days.

4.

CONSIDER YOURSELF IN INTENSIVE CARE

- Something catastrophic has happened in your life. Something assaulting to the very core of your being. Something excruciatingly painful.
- Your spirit has been deeply injured. Just as your body could not be expected to recover immediately from a brutal attack, neither can your psyche.
- Imagine that you've suffered a severe physical injury and are in the hospital's intensive care unit. Your friends and family surround you with their presence and love. They help support you as you heal. Your body rests and recovers.
- This is the kind of care you need and deserve right now: Physical and emotional intensive care. The blow you have suffered is no less devastating than this imagined physical injury. Allow others to take care of you. Ask for their help. Give yourself as much resting time as possible. Take time off work. Let household chores slide. In the early weeks and months after the death, don't expect—indeed, don't try—to carry on with your normal routine.

CARPE DIEM:

Close your eyes and imagine yourself in emotional as well as physical intensive care. Where are you? What kind of care are you receiving? From whom? Arrange a weekend of the emotional, physical, and spiritual intensive care that you need the most.

5.

BE COMPASSIONATE WITH YOURSELF

- The journey through grief is a long and difficult one, and your body is going to keep reminding you of this reality. Be compassionate with yourself as you encounter painful thoughts and feelings as well as physical aches and pains. Allow yourself to think and do whatever you need to think and do to survive. Give sustenance to your body to help survive this journey.
- Don't judge yourself or try to set a particular course for healing. There is no single, right way to grieve, and there is no set timetable.
- Let your journey be what it is. And let yourself—your new, grieving self—be who you are.
- If others judge you or try to direct your grief in ways that seem hurtful or inappropriate, ignore them. You are the only expert of your grief. Usually people are well-intentioned, but they may lack insight. See if you can muster some compassion for them, too.

CARPE DIEM:

What are you beating yourself up about these days? If you have the energy (and you don't always), address the problem head-on. If you can do something about it, do it. If you can't, try to be self-forgiving.

6.

UNDERSTAND THE DIFFERENCE BETWEEN GRIEF AND MOURNING

- Grief is the constellation of internal thoughts and feelings we have when someone loved dies. Grief is the weight in the chest, the churning in the gut, the unspeakable thoughts and feelings.
- Mourning is the outward expression of grief. Mourning is crying, journaling, creating artwork, talking to others about the death, telling the story, speaking the unspeakable.
- Everyone grieves when someone loved dies, but if we are to heal, we must also mourn. If you grieve but don't mourn, your body will keep telling you it is under distress.
- Many of the ideas in this book are intended to help you care for your body as you mourn, as you express the grief outside of yourself. Over time, and with the support of others, to mourn is to heal.

CARPE DIEM:

Ask yourself this: Have I truly been mourning the death of my loved one, or have I restricted myself to grieving?

7.

TAKE GOOD CARE OF YOURSELF

- Good self-care is nurturing and necessary for mourners, yet it's something many of us completely overlook. This entire book is devoted to encouraging you to take good care of yourself.

- You'll find more details on each of these self-care musts throughout this book, but for now:

    - Try very hard to eat well and get adequate rest. Lay your body down two to three times a day for 20-30 minutes, even if you don't sleep. You may not care very much about eating well right now, and you may sleep poorly. But taking care of yourself is truly one way to fuel healing and to begin to embrace life again.
    - Drink at least five to six glasses of water each day, more if you can. Dehydration can compound feelings of fatigue and disorientation.
    - Exercise not only provides you with more energy, it can give you focused thinking time. Take a 20-minute walk every day. Or, if that seems too much, a five-minute walk. But don't over-exercise; your body needs extra rest, as well.

- Now, more than ever, you need to allow time for you.

CARPE DIEM:

Are you taking a multivitamin? If not, now is probably a good time to start.

8.

BE KIND TO YOUR BODY

- As you have probably discovered, the loss of someone loved can take a toll on your body, potentially causing a multitude of physical problems. Do you feel tension in your body right now?
- The physical problems encountered from grief can include physical and emotional exhaustion, uncontrollable crying, trouble sleeping, heart palpitations, and headaches.
- There may be a worsening of chronic conditions such as high blood pressure, eczema, or asthma. Other chronic conditions can also be made worse when you are experiencing the need to mourn and forget to take your needed medicines.
- These physical effects are not inevitable, but in order to nurture your body, you may have to take a step back, slow down, and look at your physical needs. You may need to take time away from work and focus on clearing your mind. You must be kind to yourself by supplying your body with the good nutrition, water, rest, and exercise that you need.

CARPE DIEM:

Do one nice thing for your body today. Consider a walk, a healthy meal, a warm cup of tea, or simply a hot bath.

9.

MOVE TOWARD YOUR GRIEF, NOT AWAY FROM IT

- Our society teaches us that emotional pain is to be avoided, not embraced, yet it is only in moving toward our grief that we can be healed.
- The only way to get to the other side is through.
- Be suspicious if you find yourself thinking you are "doing well" since the death. Sometimes "doing well" means you are avoiding your pain or you're simply experiencing the natural numbness of grief. Our bodies may remind us of our inner turmoil through fatigue, headaches, and other symptoms. Listen to your body's wisdom.
- Of course, it is necessary to dose yourself with your grief. Sometimes you will need to distract yourself from the pain. But in general, you should feel that you're moving toward your grief and an understanding and acceptance of it.

CARPE DIEM:

Today, talk to someone else who cared about your loved one. Share your thoughts and feelings with him openly and encourage him to do the same. Support each other in your grief.

10.

CONSIDER YOUR OWN WELLNESS

- Wellness is defined as the pursuit of optimal health through responsible behavior choices. It goes beyond the conventional definition of health—the absence of disease or being "not sick."
- The dimensions of wellness include physical health, emotional health, cognitive health, social health, and spiritual health.
- It is important to monitor your own wellness as you move through your grieving process. Take action and seek help whenever you find that one or more of your wellness dimensions is suffering.

CARPE DIEM:

Make an inventory of how you are doing in each of your wellness dimensions: physical, emotional, cognitive, social, and spiritual. Take steps to improve yourself in one of these dimensions by using the ideas in this book

11.

INVENTORY YOUR PHYSICAL HEALTH HABITS

- Once you are through the initial survival phase of grief, you may want to take time to make an inventory of your health habits. Choose good habits to keep you healthy through your grieving period. Diet and exercise are a good place to start. Small changes may be easier to make than big ones. But first take a look at both your good and bad habits in diet, exercise, smoking, alcohol use, and hydration.

- A healthy diet has many benefits. Heart disease, certain cancers, stroke, diabetes, and damage to your arteries can be linked to what you eat. By making healthier food choices, you can also lower your cholesterol and lose weight.

- Many Americans carry too much weight, which can increase your risk for high blood pressure, high cholesterol, diabetes, heart disease, stroke, certain cancers, gallbladder disease, and arthritis in the weight-bearing joints (such as the spine, hips, and knees). A diet high in fiber and low in fat and simple carbohydrates (including sugar), along with regular exercise, can help you lose weight and keep it off.

- Exercise can help prevent heart disease, high blood pressure, diabetes, osteoporosis, and depression. It can also guard against colon cancer, stroke, and back injury. You will feel better and keep your weight under control if you exercise regularly. The goal is to exercise 30 to 60 minutes four to six times weekly, but keep in mind that any amount of exercise is better than none.

CARPE DIEM:

Choose one health habit and start improvement today.

12.

CHOOSE A PRIMARY CARE DOCTOR

- Take care of your medical needs. Having a primary care doctor who knows your medical history and takes care of the majority of your medical problems is important to your long-term health. This can be a family doctor, an internal medicine doctor, or, if you are a woman, a gynecologist. This relationship with a doctor is especially important during your time of grief when, with stress, you may have more symptoms and be more susceptible to medical problems.
- A primary care doctor should create a caring relationship with you. He or she should get to know you, listen, and help make the right healthcare decisions. Be sure to let your doctor know about the death and the grief that you feel.
- Family doctors are trained to care for you in all areas of medicine, and can diagnose and treat a full range of most problems. They also know when to bring in a trusted specialist if the problem is more complicated. They can listen and support you through your grief process.

CARPE DIEM:

If you don't already have a primary care doctor or if you haven't seen one lately, make an appointment to see one in the next two weeks.

13.

TAKE YOUR MEDICINE

- You haven't been getting enough sleep. It's hard to concentrate. You may be so distracted that you can't remember if you have taken your prescribed medication or not. The grief of loss can be all-consuming. But missing doses of medication can be a problem if you have chronic medical issues, especially those like diabetes, high blood pressure, or heart disease, which are conditions that often need close control.
- Other chronic conditions can worsen during your period of grief, so it is important to follow the instructions of your prescribed medicines in order to keep your medical problems under control. This is a vital part of self-care. Many conditions, such as high blood pressure, may not alert you with symptoms if you stop your medicine, but can do silent damage to your body.
- Taking your medicines may well be a part of your focus on survival, just like eating good foods, drinking water, and rest. It is important to slow down and be sure you are doing what you need to do to get through each day. Taking care of your body by taking needed medications is one relatively easy way to care for yourself.

CARPE DIEM:

Put your medications into a pill dispenser, and put the dispenser in a place where you will see it each morning.

14.

RECOGNIZE THAT YOUR MIND AND BODY INTERACT

- You feel intense stress from your loss and are anxious and upset, but because mind and body are interlinked, you may also feel physical symptoms and develop physical problems. However, these bodily problems are not inevitable, and if you take steps to take care of yourself, you can avoid them.

- Anxiety is common during grieving, and because anxiety activates the sympathetic nervous system, you may experience a racing pulse, sweating, poor sleep, and even loss of appetite. This is a part of our body's hardwired "fight or flight" response, which protected us when we were attacked by animals in ancient times. However, if you take time, slow down, and focus on ways to relax and use your body's natural relaxation abilities, you can bring your anxiety level back down.

- In your grief, you may turn to alcohol, recreational drugs, or prescription drugs at this stressful time to numb your feelings or control physical symptoms. Unfortunately, these substances can compound your problems. Natural relaxation techniques have many fewer side effects than drugs or alcohol.

- Finding healthier ways to control the intense stress and anxiety may also help alleviate many of the bodily symptoms you are experiencing. Taking the time to learn and practice relaxation techniques is an important way for you to find relief from both mental and physical symptoms.

CARPE DIEM:

Practice a relaxation technique such as walking, meditating, or taking a hot bath consistently for at least one week. Make note of the mental or physical symptoms that improve with this practice.

15.

BEFRIEND EIGHT UNIVERSAL HEALING PRINCIPLES

- Eight healing principles, used in the majority of cultures, can help sustain your physical, emotional, cognitive, social, and spiritual well-being. Explore the list below and note which of the universal principles you are embracing and which you are neglecting.

SUPPORT HEALTH AND WELL-BEING	NONSUPPORTIVE OF HEALTH AND WELL-BEING
Balanced diet	Unbalanced diet
Daily and weekly exercise	Lack of exercise
Time for fun, play, and laughter	Loss of humor and lack of fun and play
Music, sonics and chanting	Lack of music, sonics, and chanting
Love, touch, and support systems	Lack of love, touch, and support systems
Engaged in interests, hobbies and and creative purposes	Lack of interests, hobbies, and creative purposes
Nature, beauty, and healing environments	Lack of nature, beauty, and healing environments
Faith and belief in the supernatural	Lack of faith and belief in the supernatural

CARPE DIEM:

Make a commitment to rebalance those areas that are not supportive to your overall well-being. Get out a piece of paper right now and write out an "action plan for creating balance."

16.

BE KIND TO YOUR NERVOUS SYSTEM

- With your loss, you may feel tired and lethargic. Your nervous system is on overload, which can result in feelings of physical exhaustion. Difficulty sleeping can contribute to this overall fatigue.
- The death of someone in your life sets off a powerful stress response in your body, with release of high levels of natural, body-produced steroids and a heightened state of awareness in the nervous system. The autonomic nervous system controls the body's readiness for action in this manner.
- You can help respond to this nervous overload by giving yourself permission to slow down and take the time you need to allow your nervous system to quiet. You may first just need some time away and solitude to feel your feelings. You may need to lighten your workload and social commitments. After this, you may move forward with regular exercise, stress reduction, good nutrition, and adequate sleep and rest.

CARPE DIEM:

When you are in inner turmoil, make an assessment and take one step to quiet your nervous system. Early in the process, this may be just solitude, meditation, or prayer. Later you may consider exercise or more active stress-reduction techniques.

17.

UNDERSTAND THE ANXIETY YOU FEEL

- The fight or flight response—your body's reaction to stress—is like a fire engine responding to a call. Just like the rapid preparation of a firefighting crew, your body quickly prepares for an emergency by raising your blood pressure, breathing rate, and speed of metabolism. Muscle tension increases, and your brainwaves become more intense. There is a 300 to 400 percent increase of blood flow to the muscles of the arms and legs, to prepare your body to fight or flee. You are ready for physical action. The stress of grief can bring on this reaction, and your bodily symptoms are often a result of this response.

- Even though stress triggers this survival circuitry, most of the stresses we face in our lives are in essence false alarms, because we can't solve our problems by fighting or running. But this kneejerk reaction that has protected humans for millions of years is ingrained in our physiology. Because we do not normally react to stressful situations with physical exertion, we do not burn up the energy we have mobilized and may suffer a wide variety of negative repercussions in our bodies.

- Not only do our bodies respond negatively to stress, which increases our risk for heart disease through elevated blood pressure and enlarged and strained hearts, but elevated levels of chemical messengers like adrenaline and noradrenaline can contribute to higher levels of anxiety, depression, anger, and hostility.

CARPE DIEM:

Take time to assess your levels of racing thoughts and anxiety. Try reducing your physiologic stress through simple exercises such as walking, gardening, or bicycling.

18.

SEEK SAFETY AND COMFORT

- After a traumatic experience like a death, it's natural to feel vulnerable, unsafe, and anxious. Your nervous system is telling your brain that the world isn't a safe place right now. Something horrible has happened, and you may naturally think that it could happen again.
- To overcome your trauma, you must locate yourself among people and in places that make you feel safe. If this means moving in with a friend or relative temporarily, that's OK. You need to have those loved ones who provide intensive care around to help support you.
- What calms and comforts you? Taking a walk? Cuddling with someone you love? Hugging your pet? Relaxing in the tub? Yoga or meditation or prayer? Identify activities that soothe you, and turn to them when your anxiety is high.
- You will not be able to mourn if you feel unsafe or overly anxious. Seek safety and comfort first, then you can begin to slowly embrace your grief.

CARPE DIEM:

Let someone else take care of you today. It's normal and natural to need help with the activities of daily living in the early days and weeks after a death.

19.

CRY

- Tears are a natural cleansing and healing mechanism. It's OK to cry. In fact, it's good to cry when you feel like it. It lets the anxiety of your body wash out with your tears. What's more, tears are a form of mourning; they are sacred!
- On the other hand, don't feel bad if you are not crying a lot. Not everyone is a crier. Some people do not feel the need to cry, especially as death grows more distant. The inability to cry is not a weakness.
- You may find that those around you are uncomfortable with your tears. As a society we're not so good at witnessing others in pain.
- Explain to your friends and family that you need to cry right now and that they can help by allowing you to express your grief.
- You may find yourself crying at unexpected times or places. If you need to, excuse yourself and retreat to somewhere private. Better yet, befriend your tears and feel no sense of shame or need to conceal your authentic feelings.

CARPE DIEM:

If you feel like it, have a good cry today. Find a safe place to embrace your pain and cry as long and hard as you want.

20.

BE AWARE OF GRIEF "OVERLOAD"

- Sometimes people (maybe you) experience more than one loss in a short period of time. A traumatic event may result in many deaths. A child's death may be closely followed by a parent's death. Or an accident may claim the lives of more than one loved one.

- Other types of losses—job changes, divorce, illness, children leaving home—can also occur on top of death loss.

- When this happens, you may be at risk for "grief overload." Your ability to cope may be stretched beyond its limits. You may think of nothing but death. You may have physical symptoms, like headaches, fatigue, and poor sleep. You may feel torn, grieving one death this minute and another death the next. You may feel like you're going crazy.

- Rest assured, you are not going crazy. You are, however, in need of special care. You must try to find ways to cope with all the stress yet still find the time and focus you need to mourn. Reach out to others for help. You cannot get through this alone. See a counselor, if only to help you survive the early weeks after the deaths. Join a support group. Start a grief journal. Be proactive in getting help for yourself and mourning openly. Remember, you have special needs right now and deserve support.

CARPE DIEM:

If you're grief overloaded right now, sit down and make a list of five things you can do immediately to help offload some of your stress and help your physical symptoms. Make it a point to take action on these five things today.

21.

FIND TIME TO RELAX

- After a death there can be many demands on your time and energy. Have you taken any time to relax today? Relaxing in many forms can trigger your body's natural relaxation, which can quiet your mind and body.
- The cells of your body use oxygen from the air you breathe to burn the nutrients that you eat in a process called metabolism. The hallmark feature of the body's relaxation response is a significant decrease in the body's oxygen consumption and a downturn of metabolism.
- The body responds to techniques that elicit the relaxation response by downshifting your metabolism and lowering your energy expenditure. Along with this metabolic decrease there is a slowing of heart and breathing rates, a lessening in muscle tension, and an increase in slow brainwaves.
- This relaxation response is exactly opposite of the fight or flight response, in which the body up-shifts from its at-rest metabolic rate.

CARPE DIEM:

Take time to relax and see if you can elicit your relaxation response.
Try some deep breathing, take a walk, or stretch your muscles.
Can you make your heart rate slow? Do you feel calmer?

22.

CALM YOUR BODY

- Do a scan of your body. Do your muscles feel tight around the temples? Do you have a headache? Are your neck muscles knotted? With the stress of loss, you can have physical symptoms from the muscle tension you feel.
- With practice, you can tell your body to relax with simple mental cues or techniques. Calming the tenseness in your body by relaxation techniques can allow you to feel better and prevent harm to your body.
- First, sit comfortably in a quiet place and clear your mind; a few deep breaths may help. Mentally focus on your left hand and repeat to yourself, "My left hand feels warm and heavy." Keep doing this until your left hand does feel heavier and warmer.
- Repeat the exercise using your right hand. Then sequentially focus on your arms, legs, feet, and other body parts until your whole body feels relaxed.
- When you are done, stand up slowly, stretch your arms over your head, and take one last, deep cleansing breath.

CARPE DIEM:

Try this body-calming technique today. Make a mental note to feel the difference in the tenseness of your body before and after.

23.

TRY PROGRESSIVE MUSCLE RELAXATION

- Sometimes in dealing with your grief, you can become so stressed and "geared up" that you're no longer sure what relaxation feels like. Progressive muscle relaxation is a technique that can actually help you feel the difference between tension and relaxation.

- First you tense a muscle and notice how that tight muscle feels, then you release the tension and pay attention to this relaxed feeling, and finally you concentrate on the difference between the two feelings.

- Start with your hand. Tighten the muscle and make a firm fist. Your muscles are tight and strained, and you may even shake a bit. You may feel tension in your hand, wrist, and lower arm. Hold the tension a few seconds before relaxing. Now release your hand, relax your fist, and let the tension slip away. Your hand may feel lighter than when it was tense, and your wrist and forearm may feel relieved of pressure.

- Notice the difference between how your hand felt when it was tensed and how it feels when you release the tension. Your hand may tingle or even feel warm when relaxed. The throbbing you felt under muscle tension should disappear when your muscle relaxes.

- It's good to try this exercise on each of the major muscle groups of the body. You can start with your hands and then progress up your arms to other muscles, or you can start the exercise at the top of the body and move from head to toe by starting with the muscles of your scalp and head, then your face, shoulders, arms, hands, chest, stomach, legs, and feet.

CARPE DIEM:

Start today, and before bedtime try progressive muscle relaxation to get your tension level down before sleep.

24.

TRY A MASSAGE

- Are your neck and shoulders or other parts of your body tight and tense from the stress of dealing with your loss? Consider a soothing massage to relax the muscle tightness and relieve the pain that you feel.

- Maybe you think of massage only as a luxury in exotic spas and upscale health clubs, but did you know that massage therapy, when combined with traditional medical treatments, is used to reduce stress and pain and promote healing in tense muscles?

- During a massage, a therapist manipulates your body's soft tissues—your muscles, skin, and tendons—using his or her fingertips, hands, and fists. Several versions of massage are available, and they are performed in a variety of settings.

- Millions of people worldwide turn to massage for relaxation, relief of stress and anxiety, and to reduce muscle soreness. Massage can also cause your body to release natural painkillers and may boost your immune system.

- Consider an occasional massage as a vital part of the ongoing care and maintenance of your body. Your doctor may be able to refer you to a professional massage therapist, and, in some cases, massage therapy may even be covered by insurance.

CARPE DIEM:

Be kind to your body and relieve your stress
by scheduling a massage today.

25.

TAKE A BUBBLE BATH

- In our hurry-up world, showers are usually the order of the day. We often don't allow time for the pleasure of taking a long, hot bubble bath. But it can relieve tension in both the mind and the body. Your body is hurting from your loss, and soothing it with a warm bath may be just what you need.
- Draw a hot, hot bath. Pour in some bath salts, oils, or bubbles. Place lit candles around the bathroom (safely!). Turn off the overhead lights.
- Soak until the water grows tepid. Clear your mind and focus on the sensation of the water lapping around you.

CARPE DIEM:

Buy bath bubbles or oils and take time this evening for a soothing bath.

26.

DON'T TAKE ON ADDITIONAL STRESS RIGHT NOW

- Your plate is full right now—emotionally, spiritually, and physically. Now is not the time to take on additional stress in the form of increased workload, new commitments, or elective life changes, among other things. Your mind, body, and spirit are not ready for more.

- If you can (and this may not always be possible), try to avoid making any major decisions for at least a year following the death. Life changes such as moving to a new house or a new city, switching jobs, or getting divorced or remarried may seem like proactive, positive steps. But often such major upheavals only compound stress and delay your mourning.

- Keep your life simple right now. Do what you need to do to get through the day. Spend your time with people you love, doing the things that give you pleasure. Eliminate or set limits with friends who drain you or make you feel worse when you're around them.

CARPE DIEM:

Is there a commitment in your life that feels like a burden right now? Maybe you can temporarily give it up. Today, look into de-stressing your schedule.

27.

CUT SOME EXISTING STRESS IF YOU CAN

- When in grief, you are often overwhelmed by all the tasks and commitments you have. Your body and mind may not be able to function well enough to keep up with your busy schedule. If you can rid yourself of some of those extraneous burdens, you'll have more time for your family and friends and for mourning and healing.
- What is it that is burdening you right now? Have your name taken off junk mail lists, ignore your dirty house, stop going to optional meetings you don't look forward to attending.
- Ask a friend to help you with running errands, getting groceries, paying bills, etc. Often your friends would like to help but don't know how. This is one practical, tangible way they can.

CARPE DIEM:

Have a family meeting and take stock of your activities calendar. Ask everyone which activities they truly want to continue and which they would be happier without. Make cuts where appropriate. Maybe you can even fill in some of the extra time you'll have with a little vacation.

28.

GET HELP WITH HOUSEKEEPING

- The many tasks of daily living can feel like too much even in the best of times. In grief, they can simply be more than you can handle.
- Cleaning may feel particularly burdensome right now. Your body and mind are turned inward, and it may be hard to have the energy to do these chores.
- Here's a thought: Don't clean this week! The health inspector probably won't shut you down, at least not for another month or two.
- You can pay someone to do the cleaning, but one of your friends might be looking for a way to help. Ask him to help with occasional cleaning.

CARPE DIEM:

Call a maid service or a friend and schedule someone to come to your house for a half-day this week. Provide her with a list of the top 10 things you'd like to have taken care of.

29.

PRACTICE JUST BEING

- Sometimes what we need most is just to "be." In our goal-oriented society, many of us have lost the knack for simply living.
- Besides, just "being" may be all that you feel up to right now. Listen to your body if you don't feel like moving. It's OK.
- If you are tense and breathing rapidly and shallowly, practice slowing down your breathing and take deeper breaths.
- Drop all your plans and obligations for today and do nothing.

CARPE DIEM:

Don't "do" anything you don't want to do for the rest of the day. Instead, listen to your inner voice. What does it want to do right now?

30.

TAKE A DEEP BREATH

- A very basic need of survival is the air we breathe. With the stress of your loss, even breathing may seem difficult. If you are anxious, you may be taking rapid, short, shallow breaths, which may cause you to feel lightheaded or dizzy.

- Simply taking a deep breath can trigger a natural relaxation response within your body. Breathing slowly and deeply is one way to "turn off" your stress reaction and "turn on" relaxation.

- By inhaling deeply and allowing your lungs to take in as much oxygen as possible, you can begin to relieve your tension. Best of all, deep breathing can be done anywhere and anytime.

- First, sit or stand and place your hands on your stomach. Inhale slowly and deeply through your nose, letting your stomach expand as much as possible. Many people are "backward breathers" and tighten their stomachs when breathing in. But by placing your hands on your stomach, you can actually feel when you are breathing properly, which will help trigger relaxation. When you have breathed in as much as possible, hold your breath for a few seconds before exhaling.

- With your hands still on your stomach, exhale slowly through your mouth, pursing your lips like you are going to whistle. By pursing your lips, you can control how fast you exhale and keep your airways open as long as possible. When your lungs feel empty, start the cycle again by inhaling and exhaling. Repeat this at least three or four times per session. See how much calmer you feel already.

CARPE DIEM:

Practice deep breathing for a few minutes three or four times daily, or whenever you begin to feel tense.

31.

SIGH

- Sighing is an expression of letting go. When we sigh, we resign ourselves to something. We accept something, though perhaps it is something we didn't want to accept. It helps release the tension in our bodies.
- In Romans 8 it says that when there are no words for our prayer, the spirits intervene and pray for us in sighs deeper than anything that can be expressed in words.
- Sigh deeply. Sigh whenever you feel like it. With each sigh, you are acknowledging that you are not in total control of your life. You are accepting what is.
- Each sigh is your prayer.

CARPE DIEM:

Right now, take a deep breath and sigh. Do this ten times in a row. How do you feel?

32.

MEDITATE

- The aim of meditation is to bring inner peace to ourselves and to the world. The world is not always a peaceful place, and with your loss, your soul is full of stress and turmoil. It is therefore essential to create positive and peaceful thoughts to bring peace to your mind. Meditation is one of the best ways to bring about transformation and nurture the natural qualities within.

- The best attitude towards meditation is patience, as the mind does not always want to focus. But by practicing regularly, you can gain a wonderful sense of yourself and feel peace. Meditation is a self-healing process, and any form of stress is a sign of tension or "dis-ease" within the mind. If we don't attend to dis-ease within the mind, we may find that chronic stress can lead to disease of the body.

- Try this simple meditation. Find a quiet room and sit comfortably. Read the following passage several times, and try to open your mind to the words and feelings within the passage.

Open my mind's eye so I may see and feel your shining light presence close to me. Give me inner strength for my stumbling feet as I battle the crowd on life's busy street. And widen the vision of my unseeing mind's eye so in passing faces I will recognize not just a stranger, unloved and unknown, but a friend with a heart and a soul that is much like mine. – Ruth Ann Mahaffey

CARPE DIEM:

Try repeating this meditation for five minutes or so daily for one week. If you have another favorite passage or prayer, try it instead. Do you feel peaceful after completing this exercise?

33.

MEDITATE TOWARDS HEALING

- If you are far enough along in your healing, and you feel comfortable with meditation, you may want to try this meditation to move yourself towards healing. Repeat these thoughts in your mind:

  "I am a peaceful soul. My aim today is to have a peaceful mind and radiate peace to every person I come into contact with."

- Try to experience the stillness of mind of a peaceful soul. As thoughts emerge in your mind, do not judge or focus on them but repeat…*"I am a peaceful soul…I am a peaceful soul…My mind is filled with peace…I radiate peace to the world…I feel the gentle waves of peace flowing across my mind."*

  "I am a being of light with peace shining like a star…I radiate peace and light to the world…The light and peace envelop me and the waves of peace and light shine from my mind like a lighthouse…I continue to radiate peace to the world as I fill my mind with peace, love, and light…Through this peace I feel love and benevolence for all souls...especially those departed."

  "I see on the screen of my mind a radiant light, and this light feels gentle and soothing…I, the peaceful soul, feel at peace with myself; this stillness of mind allows me to feel content and complete…With my light of peace I can now begin to heal…With my light of peace I can feel whole and content."

CARPE DIEM:

Try this healing meditation once a week when you first wake up in the morning until you feel the light of peace fill you so you can begin your daily journey to healing.

34.

QUIET YOUR MONKEY MIND

- Buddhists have a wonderful term for the churning mental chaos that can occur with anxiety. Literally the word "papanca" means "monkey mind." It expresses the mental racing that occurs with stress as our minds leap from thought to thought without reprieve. Our minds can resemble a monkey jumping from tree limb to tree limb as we wrestle with our thoughts. The stress of loss can bring on this state of monkey mind.

- With monkey mind, we have excess brain activity that can overload our systems, making it difficult to concentrate, to learn new things, and to fall asleep.

- To combat this monkey mind, we must use our body's natural relaxation response. Our ancestors probably called on this response unwittingly when they gazed at sunsets or stared at the horizon or other wonders of nature.

- In our busy world, it is harder to find the time to enjoy quiet and uninterrupted solace, but we can make the conscious choice to relax and quiet our minds. This becomes even more important during times of grief and loss in our lives.

CARPE DIEM:

Take ten minutes today to relax and quiet your mind, watch a sunset, meditate, or take a walk.

35.

CALM YOUR MIND WITH VISUALIZATION

- Visualization is like taking a mental vacation. It frees your mind while keeping your body in a calm state.
- To get started, pick a comfortable place to sit or lie down without a lot of distracting noise or activity. Then, picture yourself feeling warm and relaxed. Visualize a peaceful setting that you enjoy, like the beach or a mountain stream, and fill in the details in your mind.
- If you choose a tropical beach, listen to the waves on the shore as you picture the scene in your mind. Feel the sun on your face, dig your toes into the sand, and feel yourself at the beach. Now spend five or ten minutes just enjoying the sensations of your mental vacation.
- By using the power of your mind, you can take a soothing break whenever you need one. Taking these mental breaks is an important part of being able to "dose" yourself with your grief.

CARPE DIEM:

Set aside a regular time each day to take a mental vacation through visualization.

36.

BE KIND TO YOUR IMMUNE SYSTEM

- The death of someone you love can, according to researchers, have a strong effect on your immune system, and for older people the effect is even more striking.
- Loss can affect your antibody response to disease. It can also cause a decrease in the activation of protective white blood cells, which are important in fighting infection. So colds and minor infections may be more common in your time of grief, and it may take longer for you to recover. Other stressors can also affect the immune system, but bereavement has the most potent effect of all stressors on the immune system.
- However, these effects are not inescapable. By taking care of your body's basic needs—food, water, and rest—you in turn will help your immune system by giving your body the sustenance it needs.
- When you start feeling more energy, you can move forward with activities that will help keep your immune system strong, such as regular exercise, stress reduction, regular sleeping hours, and even vitamin supplements.
- Be kind to yourself in ways that will help keep your immune system strong, and you can help avoid the physical effects of grief on your body.

CARPE DIEM:

Take one step to be kind to your immune system. If you are still in shock and in the early stages of grieving, just concentrate on survival issues: food, water, and rest. If you are further along, try adding exercise or some type of stress reduction, like meditation or prayer.

37.

START THE DAY WITH A GOOD NIGHT'S SLEEP

- How is your sleep? Nothing is more essential for starting a day off than getting a good night's sleep. In your grieving, you may have trouble sleeping. In fact, on any given night, one in three people have trouble falling or staying asleep—mourning or not! In your time of grief, care for yourself by allowing time for enough sleep and listening to your body.
- A normal night of sleep consists of several distinct stages and types of sleep. Stage 1 is the twilight zone between being awake and asleep. Stage 2 sleep brings larger brain waves, and we are no longer conscious of our surroundings. In Stages 3 and 4, our brains produce slower and larger waves, referred to as delta or slow wave sleep. The "lethargy of grief" often results in sleep disturbance and the inability to get enough sleep in Stages 3 and 4.
- After about 90 minutes in the four stages of quiet sleep, the brain shifts into the more active stage characterized by rapid eye movement (REM). Brain waves during REM resemble those of waking, but the large muscles of the body cannot move. This is the time of vivid dreaming. During a typical night we spend about 25 percent of the time in REM sleep and may have four or five cycles of REM sleep. We need to have enough time in each stage of sleep for our bodies and minds to be renewed.

CARPE DIEM:

Start tomorrow off better by allowing yourself to go to bed at least eight hours before you need to get up.

38.

PRACTICE GOOD SLEEP HABITS

- Stress and sleeplessness feed on each other, and you probably are struggling to sleep right now. The more tired you are, the more difficulty you have sleeping. And the more tired you are, the less capable you are of coping with stress and the more stressful life seems.
- Exercise in the morning or afternoon, but not within three hours of bedtime. Maintain exposure to bright light during the day, and avoid bright light at night to keep your circadian (or 24-hour) rhythm intact.
- It is also important to avoid heavy meals and drinking fluids within three hours of bedtime. Avoid stimulants such as caffeine and nicotine. Even alcohol can disturb sleep.
- Buy new bedding if your mattress, pillows, sheets, and blankets need replacing.
- Create a sleep environment free of temperature extremes and disruptive noises. Avoid excessive wakeful time in bed, and follow a regular, relaxing routine before bed.

CARPE DIEM:

Consider your regular sleep routine. Allow relaxing time before bed, and keep to a regular bedtime. Start this today.

39.

GET UP WITH THE BIRDS

- The sun is a powerful symbol of life and renewal.
- When is the last time you watched the sun rise? Do you remember being touched by its beauty and power?
- Plan an early morning breakfast or walk in a location where you can see the sun rise (especially if you'll probably be awake anyway because of difficulties with sleeping!). Combining some exercise with the mind-calming experience of a sunrise can not only help your health, but improve your outlook on life. Hike to the top of a hill. Have coffee on a patio next to a lake. Let the symbolic rising of the sun lift your spirit.
- Walking at daybreak may also help you sleep better tonight.

CARPE DIEM:

Invite a friend on an early morning hike. Choose a fitting destination for watching the sun rise. Pack a brunch of hot coffee, rolls, fresh fruit.

40.

MAKE SMALL CHANGES TO KEEP YOUR DIET HEALTHY

- Good nutrition is one of the keys to good health and is important for you to consider during your time of loss, when your appetite may be either suppressed or stimulated by the stress you feel. Simple things may go a long way in keeping your diet healthy and your body strong.

- Good nutrition means regularly eating foods that have ample vitamins and minerals in them, such as fruits, vegetables, whole grains, and low-fat or nonfat diary. Making healthier, lower-fat meat and poultry choices is also a good idea.

- It may seem overwhelming to consider big dietary changes while grieving, but even very small changes can improve your health considerably. The key is to keep trying to eat the right foods, and if you have medical problems, to stay in touch with your doctor and/or nutritionist so they are aware of what you are doing.

- First, just be sure you are eating enough. Is your appetite completely suppressed? Be sure to take the time to sit down and have a hot meal even if you may not feel like eating.

- Next, look at the strong and weak points of your current diet. Do you get enough calcium? Do you eat whole grain, high-fiber foods regularly? If not, try adding these foods to your diet.

- Make small, slow changes instead of trying to make large, fast ones. Small changes will be easier to make and stick with, especially when you are overwhelmed by grief.

CARPE DIEM:

Make one small change to your diet today, such as adding more fruits and vegetables or increasing fiber to care for your body during your time of grief.

41.

EAT MORE FRUITS AND VEGGIES

- Your body needs adequate fiber, minerals, and vitamins. A simple thing you can do even when you are in survival mode is add more fruits and vegetables to your day. These foods are naturally high in vitamins as well as fiber, which is good for your digestion.
- Vitamins are important micronutrients that help keep your immune system strong and your metabolism functioning normally. Vitamins A, C, and E are antioxidants that can help counteract the stress-related chemical changes that can occur in your body during grief.
- Adding at least one to two vegetables or fruit to each meal is a simple way to ensure adequate vitamin intake. Your goal should be to eat at least five servings of vegetables and fruit daily, more if you can. Add extra fruits or vegetables as snacks. If your appetite won't allow this, then add a multivitamin with minerals daily.
- Remember, you have been torn apart, so making good food choices is an important part of your overall self-care plan. Be good to your spirit and your body—you deserve it!

CARPE DIEM:

Add at least one or two servings of fruits or vegetables to each meal.

42.

EMPLOY SOY FOR BETTER HEALTH

- Soy is a complete protein, and soy foods are rich in vitamins and minerals, including folate, potassium and, in some cases, fiber. During your time of grief, you may want to add healthy soy products to your diet to substitute for less-healthy protein sources, such as fatty red meats, to lessen your health risks.

- The FDA has recognized the cholesterol-lowering effects of soy since 1999. Consuming larger amounts of soy can lower bad cholesterol (LDL) by three percent. But studies did not show any negative effect on good cholesterol (HDL), triglycerides, or blood pressure. Most soy foods are also low in saturated fats and trans fats (types of fat that more readily cause narrowing of the arteries), and eating soy products has been shown to lower the risk of heart disease.

- Other research suggests soy may lower the risk of prostate, colon, and breast cancer as well as reduce the risk of osteoporosis, although these studies are not definitive. It was thought soy products might alleviate hot flashes from menopause, but recent studies have not verified this.

- Try adding soy milk, soy cereal, or simply soy nuts to improve your diet.

CARPE DIEM:

Add one to two servings of soy-based food to your diet daily. Choose from a variety of forms: soy milk, soy snacks, tofu, soy burgers, soy nuts, etc. Stop by a grocery store and try one today.

43.

GET THE FACTS ON FLAX

- During your time of grief, try flaxseed products to boost omega 3s, which are essential fatty acids that can help protect your heart and improve your health.
- Flaxseed comes from a blue flowering plant grown on western Canadian prairies. Flaxseed contains fiber, protein, B vitamins, and lignans, as well as essential alpha-linolenic, omega 6, and omega 3 fatty acids.
- These chemicals are important because they have qualities that can prevent diabetes and cancers and can decrease the risk of heart disease by lowering cholesterol, triglycerides, blood pressure, and plaque formation in the arteries.
- Flax has about 50 percent more omega 3 fatty acids than fish oil. Flaxseed can decrease heart disease by lowering cholesterol, triglycerides, blood pressure, and plaque formation.
- Studies have shown that people who eat oils rich in omega 3, like flaxseed oil, need less medicine for their arthritis. Omega 3 has also been found to kill certain cancer cells, and improve skin problems like eczema and psoriasis.
- You may not be able to make large changes while grieving, but adding a flaxseed capsule daily can be a simple change towards a healthier diet.

CARPE DIEM:

Try adding flaxseed oil to protein shakes or other drinks, or add a flaxseed oil supplement to take with your daily vitamin.

44.

FEEL VITAL WITH VITAMIN D

- You naturally feel fatigued in dealing with loss and may spend most of your time indoors, since you probably have little energy to go outside. If you're not exposing your skin to sunshine, you may become low in vitamin D. Recent studies have shown that many people are low in vitamin D, and indoor jobs and northern climates may elevate this risk since vitamin D is activated by exposure to sunlight.

- The chief function of vitamin D is to maintain normal levels of calcium and phosphorus by promoting their absorption in the intestinal tract. It keeps our bones strong.

- Low vitamin D levels can make you feel tired and has been linked with heart disease and high blood pressure. Vitamin D also helps regulate the immune system and may help prevent cancer.

- To be sure you are getting enough vitamin D, eat fish such as salmon or tuna, and consider vitamin D-fortified milk, soy milk, orange juice, and breads or cereals. Sunlight exposure for 10 to 15 minutes twice weekly to your face, arms, legs, or back is adequate.

- If you aren't sure you're getting enough, consider a vitamin D supplement, especially in the winter. Check with your doctor about dosages; he or she may want to check your vitamin D blood level before starting a supplement.

CARPE DIEM:

Today, spend ten minutes feeling the healing warmth of sunshine on your skin. If it's not sunny, go to the store and pick up some vitamin D-rich foods.

45.

MAKE A SIMPLE CHANGE IN COOKING OILS

- The huge assortment of vegetable cooking oils can puzzle shoppers and be overwhelming to those in mourning.
- Olive oil is probably the best all-around oil for cooking and salads. It has flavor and affordability. It is rich in monounsaturated fats, which lowers bad cholesterol (LDL), helps boost good cholesterol (HDL), and has been shown to improve heart health.
- Canola oil is an excellent, inexpensive choice when you need cooking oil with a neutral taste. Canola oil contains monounsaturated fat and also provides essential omega-3 fatty acids, both of which are good for your heart.
- Peanut oil is a good source of monounsaturated fat and vitamin E. The high smoke point makes it suitable for hot cooking such as popping popcorn, sautéing, and roasting.
- Sesame oil is available raw or roasted. This polyunsaturated oil gives a distinctive Asian tang and is especially suitable to a vegetable stir-fry or for chicken, shrimp, and lean-meat dishes.
- Nut oils in their refined forms are best for low-temperature baking. Unrefined oils add a mild nutty flavor to vinaigrettes and vegetable toppings. Walnut, hazelnut, and macadamia nut oils are a few distinctive types.

CARPE DIEM:

Pick one of the above cooking oils and try it for at least a week. Stay with it if you like the flavor.

46.

TRY FISH OIL TO FEEL BETTER

- Care for your body during your time of grief by adding fish oil to your diet. You may be too overwhelmed by grief to make a large dietary change, but adding a fish-oil tablet can be a simple thing to do to improve your health. The omega 3 essential fatty acids found in fish oil are protective to your heart. Walnuts and vegetable oils like canola, soybean, flaxseed, and olive can also be good sources of omega 3.

- The average American diet is high in omega 6 fatty acids, which are found in animal meats, and low in omega 3s. This imbalance can lead to increased plaque deposits in arteries, whereas increasing omega 3s can reduce hardening of the arteries.

- Omega 3 in fish oil has also been shown to lower blood pressure and reduce the risk of death, heart attack, dangerous abnormal heart rhythms, and strokes. Fish oil has been shown to reduce triglycerides and make small improvements in good cholesterol (HDL) levels.

- Fish oil has also been shown to reduce inflammation, which may also protect against heart disease. Many studies report improvement of arthritic symptoms with fish oil supplements, and the effects of other anti-inflammatory medicines are enhanced with fish oil.

- There are some studies that suggest fish oil may improve immune function, and having low levels of omega 3 in your body has been linked to depression.

- Many of the physical effects on your body from the stress of your loss can be minimized by adding daily fish oil tablets.

CARPE DIEM:

Try starting a daily fish oil tablet today.

47.

BE KIND TO YOUR HEART

- You are probably brokenhearted during your time of grief. However, it is important as you move through your grieving period to control your risk factors for actual heart disease. The stress of grieving may put additional strain on your heart, so it's important to reduce your risk factors for heart disease. The good news is that you have the ability to control many of these risk factors.

- There are some risk factors, such as a family history of heart disease, being male, or increasing age, which are beyond your control. However, controllable risk factors for heart disease include things like high cholesterol, high blood pressure, and a sedentary lifestyle. These are things you can influence by your behavior.

- You can control your cholesterol if it is high by eating right and exercising. Limit how much high-cholesterol and fatty foods you eat. If you're a smoker, get help to stop!

- Control your blood pressure if it is high. High blood pressure increases your risk for heart disease, stroke, and kidney disease. To control it, lose weight, exercise, eat less salt, drink less alcohol, don't smoke, and be sure to take your medicine for blood pressure if your doctor prescribes it.

- Lack of exercise speeds progression of heart disease, so consider starting some form of exercise, such as walking, to protect your heart.

CARPE DIEM:

Choose one risk factor for heart disease and
improve your behavior today.

48.

KEEP YOUR BAD CHOLESTEROL LOW

- The stress of losing someone in your life can cause a release of stress hormones that have been shown to raise cholesterol. High cholesterol can lead to hardening of the arteries, or so-called atherosclerosis. These processes are not inevitable, and you can take steps to control this rise of cholesterol through diet and exercise. After getting through the initial survival phase of grief, you may want to consider a cholesterol check.
- Both high LDL (bad cholesterol) and low HDL (good cholesterol) can raise your risk for heart disease, so it is good to look at activities that improve both.
- Low-density lipoprotein (LDL) is the damaging kind that can clog your arteries and cause heart disease. It needs to stay low. You can keep your LDL low by eating a diet low in saturated fat and cholesterol.
- If you have not had your cholesterol checked recently, arrange with your doctor to have a fasting blood sample taken. This will allow you to assess whether you need to take move active steps.
- If your bad cholesterol is high, talk with your doctor about supplements or medications that can help lower your cholesterol and reduce your risk of health problems.

CARPE DIEM:

Make arrangements to get your cholesterol checked this week.

49.

RAISE YOUR GOOD CHOLESTEROL

- As you are able to become more active during your time of grief, you may want to help improve your health by taking steps to raise your good cholesterol, or HDL. This will lower your risk for heart problems as you try to mend your broken heart from loss.
- HDL, "good cholesterol," removes excess bad cholesterol from arteries and sends it back to the liver for excretion in bile and stool. It also inhibits plaque formation within the walls of your arteries and lowers inflammation. This is why boosting HDL is a good idea.
- An HDL level lower than 40 mg/dl indicates risk for heart disease. Common contributors to low HDL include insufficient exercise, smoking, excess weight, high triglycerides (or fats in the blood), diabetes, poor diet, side effects of some medications, and genetic history.
- Aim for an HDL level of greater than 60 mg/dl. Recent findings indicate that heart disease deaths decrease four to five percent for every HDL increase of 1 mg/dl.

CARPE DIEM:

Boost your HDL today by getting 30 to 60 minutes of physical activity for as many days of the week as you can (a minimum of three or four days).

50.

CONTROL YOUR BLOOD PRESSURE

- With the burden of the stress of your loss, you may have higher blood pressure due to the activation of your sympathetic nervous system. And blood pressure is an important health parameter to consider. Even if your pressure is high, you can take the appropriate steps to control this problem before any physical issues occur. If your numbers remain high even after you've taken steps to reduce them, they can be controlled by medication your physician may prescribe.

- Some people have a family history of high blood pressure and may have an increased risk of hypertension themselves. You may not have symptoms with your high blood pressure, so it is important to have it checked.

- Your blood pressure should consistently be below 140/90—even lower if you are a diabetic, at 135/85. The top number is the systolic pressure, when your heart is beating, and the bottom number is the diastolic, which is between heartbeats.

- Start with a diet and exercise program to see if you can lower your numbers. Weight loss and a diet low in salt may also help. Be careful about drinking alcohol, which tends to raise blood pressure.

- It is essential to stay on your blood pressure medicine if a doctor has prescribed it. Don't skip doses, even when overwhelmed in your grieving process.

CARPE DIEM:

Have your blood pressure checked today.

51.

CATCH UP ON PREVENTIVE HEALTH MAINTENANCE

- Keep your shots up to date. Adults need a tetanus-diphtheria booster every 10 years. Your doctor may substitute the Td booster with one Tdap booster, which also protects against pertussis (whooping cough). You should consider a flu shot each year, and those over 65 should have a pneumonia vaccine (younger if you have chronic disease such as diabetes, heart disease, or asthma).
- Ask your doctor about cancer screenings. Adults over 50 should be checked for colorectal cancer, usually with a colonoscopy. Men over 50 should discuss with their doctor the risks and benefits of being screened for prostate cancer.
- If you are a woman, check your breasts. Breast cancer is the second most common cause of death for women. Have your doctor check your breasts every one to two years until you are 40. After age 40, have a yearly clinical exam and a mammogram.
- Women should also get regular Pap smears, which detect cervical cancer. Pap smears should be done when women start having sex or by age 18. You will need them yearly until you have had at least three normal Pap tests. After this, you should have them at least every three years.
- Men should do regular testicular self-exams. Testicular cancer is a disease that occurs most often in men in their twenties and thirties. Caught early, it is a very curable form of cancer.

CARPE DIEM:

Check with your doctor for any needed health screenings.

52.

DRINK WATER

- During your bereavement, it is important to drink plenty of water to stay healthy. This is essential, since your body is about 60 percent water and needs constant replenishment. Every system in your body depends on water. While in grief, your body is turned down and focusing on your inward feelings, and you may not feel thirsty. Remind yourself to drink adequate water to keep your body hydrated.

- Lack of water can lead to dehydration, a condition that occurs when there is not enough water in your body to carry on normal functions. Even mild dehydration of one to two percent loss of body weight can sap your energy and make you tired. This can compound the fatigue you already feel with grief.

- Signs and symptoms of dehydration include excess thirst, fatigue, headache, dry mouth, little or no urination, muscle weakness, dizziness, and lightheadedness.

- Every day you lose water through sweating (noticeable and unnoticeable), exhaling, urinating, and bowel movements. You need to replace this loss daily by consuming beverages and foods that contain water. Other factors like exercise, the environment (including heat and humidity), and illnesses or health conditions may influence your water needs.

- How much water do you need? At least five eight-ounce cups, and some people advise up to eight cups a day to maintain good hydration.

- Caring for yourself by keeping hydrated can allow you to focus on working through your grief.

CARPE DIEM:

Start today by drinking at least five eight-ounce cups of water daily.

53.

LIMIT SWEET DRINKS

- Fluids are important to keep your body functioning normally during the stress of grief. However, in our society we tend to indulge in too many sweet, caffeinated drinks, which may only make your bodily symptoms of grief worse. To avoid the swings of blood sugar during your time of grief, consider limiting soda and sweet drinks. (Besides, at more than 150 calories per 12-ounce can, the number of calories and pounds from soda quickly add up.) As you emerge from your survival period, you may want to consider eliminating soda and sweet drinks entirely.

- According to studies, diet soda drinkers gain about as much weight as with regular pop. The sweet taste may stimulate the craving for other sweets and carbohydrates, and those drinking diet soda have a 44 percent greater risk for metabolic syndrome (which is a cluster of symptoms that put you at higher risk for heart disease and diabetes).

- Pop calories are "empty" calories, since they contain no other nutritional benefits and do not contain vitamins and minerals. Carbonation (the fizziness) is achieved by using phosphates, which can bind to calcium in your diet, thereby reducing calcium absorption and leading to a weakening of bones.

- Since pop is carbonated and often contains caffeine, it may cause or aggravate stomach acid and reflux. The caffeine may make your sleep problems worse too.

- Your pancreas can become overworked, releasing insulin because of the rapid spike in blood sugar from sugary drinks. This can eventually lead to diabetes in those who are genetically prone.

CARPE DIEM:

Set a deadline to stop or cut back on soda intake. Try substituting water flavored with a slice of lemon or lime for these sugary drinks.

54.

LIMIT YOUR ALCOHOL INTAKE

- In your dark days of grief, it may be easy to turn to alcohol to numb the pain. However, drinking alcohol while you are grieving puts you at risk for addiction. Drinking alcohol can easily get out of control if you use it to try to numb the pain of your loss.

- If you do not drink, now is not the time to start. There are healthy limits to alcohol intake, and if you decide to continue to drink during your grief, it is important to stay within these limits.

- Alcohol does have some health benefits, but these are quickly replaced by greater dangers at higher amounts. Studies show positive health effects for up to two drinks a day for men and one drink a day for women. One drink is equal to one can of beer (12 ounces), a four-ounce glass of wine, or a shot glass (one ounce) of liquor. But alcohol is a double-edged sword. If you are tempted and can't control having more than these daily limits during your grief, remove the alcohol from your house and seek support from a physician or counselor.

CARPE DIEM:

Be honest about your alcohol intake. If it is above healthy limits, make a plan to talk to a physician or counselor today.

55.

TEA-WISE, GO GREEN

- The Chinese have known about the medicinal benefits of green tea since ancient times. It has been used to treat many physical ailments for more than 4,000 years.
- Green tea has long been used in Asia for its calming effects in "tea ceremonies." But green tea has also been shown in recent studies to have positive effects on the immune system and reduce infection rates. It has also been shown to prevent heart disease by lowering bad cholesterol (LDL) and raising good cholesterol (HDL). It even has a cancer-reducing effect.
- The secret of green tea is its powerful antioxidants, which have been shown to lower cholesterol, slow cancer cell growth, and inhibit the formation of blood clots. This reduction of blood clotting is how green tea reduces heart attacks and strokes. Other types of tea do not have the same types or amounts of these beneficial chemicals.
- Make a simple change by adding green tea to your life during your grief. This simple act will help you care for your mind and body and add a reassuring ritual to your life as you experience the hard work of mourning.

CARPE DIEM:

Start a daily regimen of taking time to relax, clear your mind, and have a cup of warm, soothing green tea.

56.

STOP SMOKING

- With the stress of grief, you may turn to bad habits such as smoking for relief. If you are smoking, consider reducing the number of cigarettes daily. Pick a good time to try to quit. The period of initial shock after the death is not a good time. However, as you recover and work your way through your grief, remember there is no one single behavior change that will improve your long-term health more than quitting smoking. The sooner you quit, the better.
- Heart disease, lung cancer, chronic bronchitis, and emphysema are all associated with smoking. Cancer of the mouth and throat are associated with chewing tobacco.
- More preventable illnesses, such as emphysema, cancers, and heart disease, are caused by tobacco use than by anything else.
- Your doctor may write you a prescription for medication that can be useful in stopping smoking, and there are over-the-counter medications as well. Make a well-thought-out plan of how you will quit, and then set a quit date. Be sure to line up support for yourself in getting through this difficult time. Ex-smokers are often good supporters. There are also many online and telephone support services, such as Quitline, that can help you as you quit.

CARPE DIEM:

If you smoke, make a plan for stopping and set a quit date today.

57.

RELAX BY STRETCHING

- As we've said, one of your natural physical responses to stress is muscle tension. An easy way to combat this muscle tightness is to do stretching exercises for the area in which people often carry their stress—the neck and shoulders. You can do this at home or at breaks at work. Check with your physician first if you have chronic neck or shoulder problems.

- Head turn: Stand or sit erect. Keep your back straight. Now turn your head slowly to the right as far as it will comfortably go. Hold that position to the count of five. Return to the normal position and repeat this procedure to the left. Repeat both ways five times.

- Chin tuck and lift: Stand erect, and slowly lower your chin, trying to touch your chest, as far as it will comfortably go. Hold for a count of five. Slowly raise your head back, looking up to the ceiling. Do not force or strain during the exercise. Hold the position for a count of five. Return to normal position and repeat five times.

- Lateral tilt: Stand or sit erect. Slowly bend your head to the side, bringing your left ear to the left shoulder. Hold the position for a count of five. Return to normal position and repeat this to the right shoulder. Repeat both sides five times.

- Head roll: Slowly and evenly roll your head clockwise in a wide circle. Do the same sequence counterclockwise. Repeat three times.

- Shoulder shrug: Stand or sit erect. Inhale deeply and slowly. Lift your shoulders up towards your ears. Now pull your shoulders back as far as possible. Then rotate back to normal position and exhale. Repeat this 20 times.

CARPE DIEM:

Set aside a few minutes every day to do one or more of these stretches. Do your muscles feel looser when you are done?

58.

START AN EXERCISE PROGRAM

- Increased exercise can help with stress management during your time of loss. And once you have moved beyond simple survival mode, you may be ready to begin a more aggressive exercise program. Increased physical activity can lead to a longer life and improved health. It also curbs your appetite and burns more calories. Regular exercise helps protect your organs and strengthens your muscles, bones, and blood flow as you age.

- Increased physical activity can benefit almost everyone. Most people can begin gradual moderate exercise. If there is a reason you may not be able to exercise, ask your doctor before you begin. In particular, you should talk to your doctor if you have heart trouble, high blood pressure, or arthritis, or if you have dizziness or chest pains with exercise.

- Exercises that increase your heart rate and move large muscles (like arms and legs) are the best kind. Choose an activity that you like and will enjoy doing. Walking is very popular and requires no special equipment. Other good exercises include swimming, biking, jogging, aerobics, and dancing.

- Taking the stairs instead of the elevator or walking instead of driving may also be good ways to start being more active. Walking, sports, gardening, and all physical chores count toward an exercise minimum of 30 minutes daily, even when done in ten-minute increments.

- Start off by exercising three or more times a week for 20 minutes or more, and work up to 30 minutes four to six times a week.

CARPE DIEM:

If you are starting to feel better and are beyond simple survival, find a physical activity you enjoy and start an exercise program today.

59.

TAKE A WALK

- Loss can be overwhelming, and in order to deal with these overwhelming emotions and normalize your stress hormones, walking can offer relief for both mind and body. It's easy, and even early in mourning, when you are very fatigued, you may still be able to summon enough energy to walk.
- Walking can be an aerobic activity and can do many healthy things for your body, including raising good cholesterol and lowering the risk for heart disease and stroke.
- Pick comfortable shoes, start at short distances, and choose pleasant, scenic areas in which to walk. Parks with beautiful natural areas may soothe your grieving soul during your walks.
- Use the time spent walking to clear your mind from the anxiety and pain you may feel in trying to deal with your loss. Try to just "be" and not think about stressful things while you walk. Walking can be good for both your mind and body, and can allow you to use up the stress hormones and adrenaline your body has released.

CARPE DIEM:

Clear your mind and help your body by taking a walk today.

60.

START A WEIGHT-TRAINING PROGRAM

- Maintaining or improving your strength can help you literally and figuratively feel stronger as you deal with your loss.
- Increasing your muscle mass will improve your metabolic rate, since muscle burns more calories than fatty tissue. You burn more calories just sitting when you have a greater percentage of muscle in your body. This can help you reach and maintain a lower weight.
- Weight lifting can cause serious injury if done improperly, however, so if you have never lifted weights, it is important that you find an instructor who can teach you good lifting techniques. A high school coach or athletic trainer at a health club can help. The National Strength and Conditioning Association (ncsa-lift.org) may also be able to recommend a qualified coach in your area.
- For most people, starting with light weights and doing more repetitions is an easier and safer way to begin. Generally, lifting about three times a week is the best way to improve your strength, since lifting daily may not allow your muscles time to repair and grow.
- With your instructor's help, decide on goals for your weight-training program. Your goals will depend on your age, physical maturity, and the specific reasons you may have for lifting weights.

CARPE DIEM:

Consider whether a strength program might help you feel stronger in your time of grief. If you are moving from survival mode to a more active one, start a program by contacting a trainer today.

61.

TRY BIKING FOR BODY AND MIND

- For exercise as well as mind-body connection, consider riding a bicycle during your bereavement. Who didn't love the feeling of riding a bike as a kid? It was totally freeing, and bike riding kept us lean and healthy. As an adult, bike riding offers many benefits to the body and can help you feel like a kid again.
- It goes without saying that bike riding is very beneficial for the health of your heart, since everyone needs about 30 minutes of aerobic exercise daily. Bicycling is kind to the joints, too, and if you have joint problems, biking can offer exercise without pain. The motion of pedaling is fluid rather than abrupt and puts less stress on joints.
- A bike with several speeds will allow you to increase your work as your fitness improves. Begin by riding at an easy speed, over even ground. As you improve, you can increase your speed and try more challenging terrain. It is important to wear a helmet to protect yourself from injury, and if you have not ridden in a long time, be sure to start slowly in a safe area.
- Cycling can help maintain strength and coordination. The pedaling motion can increase circulation to your legs and strengthen your leg muscles. But remember to check with your doctor to be sure this type of exercise is safe for you. If you have not ridden a bike in years, be sure to start slowly, and don't forget your helmet!

CARPE DIEM:

Feel like a kid again and try bicycling today.

62.

TAKE A SPIN

- When it's too cold to bike outdoors, try a spinning class. Spinning bikes are specially-made stationary bicycles that more closely resemble the experience of actually riding a bike. If you are beyond the simple survival stage of grieving, this may be a good way to get started exercising.

- If you think biking indoors is boring, you haven't been to a good spin class. With a motivational instructor, great music, and a dynamic workout, spin classes can get far more out of you than pedaling alone on a stationary bike.

- The instructor leads the exercises and keeps the focus, but you decide how hard to push. It's important to start slowly if you haven't been exercising, and check with your doctor if you have chronic heart or lung problems.

- Use your instructor as a resource. Tell her about your goals and even request workouts or music. Try wearing cycling shoes. Clipping into the pedals gives you more control, makes you more efficient, and works both sides of your legs—your hamstrings as well as your quads. When you start, it's important to pace yourself. A heart-rate monitor will help you keep your effort in the right range. It is also important to stay hydrated. Spin classes can be intense, so keep a water bottle within arm's reach and drink often.

- Don't be afraid to get into it. Relax, enjoy the music, and interact with the class. Bring a friend to class to make sure you go and to keep it fun. Spinning is an excellent way of helping your mind and body relieve the stress of your grief.

CARPE DIEM:

Find a spin class in your community today.

63.

DIVE INTO SWIMMING

- Swimming is not only good exercise, it's a lifetime sport that benefits not only the body but the whole person.
- Regular swimming builds endurance, muscle strength, and cardiovascular fitness. It can serve as cross-training for other types of workouts, or it can be your main source of exercise. Kickboard workouts, water aerobics, pool running, or a regular swimming workout can give you a great exercise session without the weight of your body pounding you with each move.
- Swimming is a unique exercise that works the whole body and improves conditioning, strength, and endurance as well as posture and flexibility. Your cardiovascular system in particular benefits because swimming improves your body's use of oxygen without overworking your heart. As you become fitter and are able to swim longer, your resting heart rate and respiratory rate will be reduced, making blood flow to the heart and lungs more efficient.
- Swimming tones your upper and lower body because you're using almost all of your major muscle groups. There is a low risk of injury because there is little stress on your bones, joints, and connective tissue due to the buoyancy reducing the stress on your body.
- The rhythmic exercise of swimming can calm your mind and help you with the overwhelming stress of grief that you may feel.

CARPE DIEM:

Start a regular swimming or pool-workout session today.

64.

SAY YES TO YOGA

- Yoga is an ancient form of exercise, over 3,000 years old, that originated in India. Yoga strengthens you physically, emotionally, and spiritually. Many traditions acknowledge that being on a spiritual path is like being a warrior. Practicing yoga can help you become a peaceful warrior and inspire your capacity to authentically mourn.

- Yoga has elements of ancient teachings that connect mind and body in an exercise form involving postures (asanas), breathing techniques (pranayama), and meditation. The breathing techniques or purifications can enhance inner tranquility. Yoga teaches long, slow, deep breaths, which help get oxygen to your cells and can help center you and remind you to nurture your spiritual life. Yogic breathing infuses your body with prana, or energy.

- Yoga means union or wholeness. If you are new to yoga, start with a beginner class and an instructor who can individualize the techniques to your needs.

- Yoga can improve balance, flexibility, and strength. Proponents feel it even has an anti-aging effect and can improve concentration and endurance.

- Mentally, yoga has many positive effects, including decreasing anxiety and depressive symptoms, improving mood and memory, and allowing people to feel more self-actualized and at ease with who they are. These mind and body benefits will help you as you move through your grief.

CARPE DIEM:

Check to see if any therapeutic yoga classes are available in your area and try one today.

65.

TRY TAI CHI

- Originally developed in China as a form of self-defense, tai chi (pronounced "ty chee") is a graceful form of exercise that has existed for some 2,000 years. Practiced regularly, tai chi can help you reduce your stress and can strengthen and nurture your body and spirit in your time of grief. It is based on postures that get your "good" energy flowing and resist "negative" energy.
- Tai chi is often described as "meditation in motion" because it promotes serenity through gentle movements, helping to connect the mind and the body. Tai chi has more than 100 possible movements and positions. The intensity of tai chi varies with the particular style, although all have rhythmic patterns of breathing and moving. When you are physically, emotionally, and spiritually healthy, your life force, or "chi," flows through you freely, and you are fully alive. When stressed by grief and other demands, your energy becomes blocked and you feel tired, depressed, and out of balance. The slow movements of tai chi calm you, inviting harmony into your body, and you feel at peace with the world.
- Although tai chi is generally safe, consider talking to your doctor if you have joint, spine, or heart problems before starting a new program.
- Although practiced in China for millennia, tai chi has been studied scientifically only recently. Health benefits may include reduced anxiety and depression, improved balance and coordination, improved sleep quality, lowered blood pressure, relieved chronic pain, and improved everyday physical functioning.

CARPE DIEM:

If you are interested in tai chi, find a qualified instructor in your area and sign up for a beginning session.

66.

PARTAKE OF PILATES

- If you need an exercise option that can quiet your mind and strengthen your body in your time of grief, try Pilates. It primarily involves strengthening the core muscles, particularly the back and abdomen as well as the hips and buttocks, using your own body weight as resistance. But it is also good for mind and spirit.

- The Pilates fitness method, which focuses on strength, flexibility, and balance, has been growing in popularity for years and is now mainstream for men and women of all shapes, ages, and fitness levels.

- You gain strength and joint flexibility in Pilates by controlling various movements through precise form and gradual progression. Concentration and breathing are emphasized for maximum effect.

- Workouts may consist of simple floor-work classes or special resistance machines. Instructors typically offer a series of 60-minute sessions working one-on-one or with small groups. Classes can be customized for groups that are older, pregnant, overweight, or even those who are super-fit.

- Ultimate benefits include a leaner physique, increased energy and stamina, and a stronger, pain-free back. Though Pilates can build core strength, additional workouts are recommended by fitness experts to round out your conditioning. However, even if you are in a survival mode of grief, Pilates can suffice to soothe your mind and body and could be a first step in healing both.

CARPE DIEM:

Check out a Pilates class in your area, and if it is appealing, try it.

67.

TAKE A HIKE TO EMBRACE NATURE

- We're lucky to have many amazing national, state, and city parks, along with breathtaking national forests and recreational areas. Many have wonderful hiking trails that are just waiting for you to embrace the healing force of nature. Take the time to care for your mind and body by embracing this natural healing during the time of your grief.
- Hiking is an aerobic exercise that can help raise good cholesterol and reduce risks for heart disease and stroke, and if done consistently, can be a great stress reducer.
- The beauty of nature tends to have its own way of allowing us to heal both mentally and physically from the losses we have endured. Seeing the wonders of nature can remind you that there is still beauty and peace in the world, even when you may continue to be struggling in your own mind from the desolation of loss.
- Allow the peace of nature to fill your mind and the movement of your body to release some of the buildup of adrenaline and stress hormones that most likely has come with the stress of your grief.

CARPE DIEM:

Pick a nearby natural area and take a hike to feel the embrace of nature today.

68.

GARDEN TO GROW THROUGH YOUR GRIEF

- Many people who love to garden find it a spiritual experience. During your time of grief, this would be a good activity to help both your body and mind. One of the most obvious benefits of gardening is the exercise involved. The beauty of it is that the hobby offers so many different levels of exercise that almost anyone can do it.

- The regular exercise that one gets from gardening or yard work has been shown to reduce the risk of heart disease and keep bodies supple and flexible. Gardening not only builds strength and cardiovascular fitness, but it can also relieve stress and provide nutritious food.

- People find peace in the garden, in part because they commune with the earth and in part from the visual beauty of their plants and flowers. Working in the garden and giving birth to growing things can bring you a sense of satisfaction and oneness with the world.

- Gardening can provide fresh fruits and vegetables and the encouragement to eat them. Fresh food tastes better (especially when you grew it), and it is better for you. In growing your own food, you have control over the pesticides and fertilizers that are used. Growing fresh herbs can add some spice to your life.

CARPE DIEM:

Plan to create a small garden in the spring of the year. Spend time nurturing each plant and every blooming flower. If you do not have the energy or desire to plant a garden, go visit one and enjoy the growth that will take place in the garden of your heart.

69.

DANCE THROUGH GRIEF INTO LIFE

- Dance has been described as a metaphor for life. In the midst of grief, dance can be a lovely way to transform your grief (your internal response) into mourning (the shared outward response). Dance invites you to merge with the music and movement even as it takes you outside of yourself and is also good for your body.

- Constanze referred to dance as dreaming with your feet. Sweetpea Tyler claimed it faces you toward heaven, whichever direction you turn. Martha Graham called it the hidden language of the soul.

- Dance is more than an aerobic physical activity, although it is terrific for your body. It is a complete mind, body, and spirit workout, and it is fun! (And God knows you need fun when in the wilderness of your grief.) Many forms of dance are forms of moving meditation. The blend of physical, emotional, and spiritual concentration invites both surrender and renewal, while at the same time transporting you into the spiritual realm of wholeness and connection to the world outside of yourself. Yes, there is magic in dance.

- Dance can transform you in ways that reawaken your "divine spark"—that which gives you meaning and purpose. Movement allows your body to heal, your mind to open, and your spirit to sing. Dance also engages you in community because you enter into a partnership that is greater than the sum of its parts. You discover that you are in constant, ever-flowing exchange with yourself, each other, and the Divine.

CARPE DIEM:

Take some dance lessons. Salsa, ballroom, ballet, tap, clogging, jazz, belly dancing? Pick one and get started today.

70.

STAY IN TOUCH WITH YOUR FEELINGS

- You will probably feel many different feelings in the coming weeks and months. You may feel, among other things, numb, angry, guilty, afraid, confused, and, of course, deeply sad. Sometimes these feelings follow each other within a short period of time, or they may occur simultaneously.

- Your body may also give you messages of distress, such as fatigue, palpitations, and disorientation, which may reflect your emotions. Your body's messages may be a clue to your emotional distress, even when you are feeling emotionally numb.

- As strange as some of these feelings seem to you, your feelings are what they are. They are not right or wrong; they simply are. Allow yourself to feel whatever it is you are feeling without judging yourself.

- Stay in touch with your feelings by leaning into them when you are ready. If you feel angry, for example, allow yourself to feel and think through this anger. Don't suppress it or distract yourself from it. Instead, acknowledge your feelings and give them voice. Tell a friend, "I feel so mad today because …" or write in your journal, "I feel such regret that…"

- Learning to name your feelings will help you tame them. As Shakespeare's Macbeth reminds us, "Give sorrow words: the grief that does not speak whispers with o'er-fraught heart, and bids it break."

CARPE DIEM:

Using old magazines, clip images that capture the many feelings you've been having since the death. Make a "feelings collage" on poster board and display it somewhere you'll be able to reflect on it.

71.

KNOW THE SIGNS OF DEPRESSION

- Depression can occur as a consequence of the stress that occurs with loss. Feeling down or blue is a normal part of grief, but if your depressed mood is severe and does not improve over time, and you have other mood symptoms as well (anger, hopelessness, irritability, etc.), then you may want to explore this with a trained professional.

- Depressive symptoms include the following:

    - Little interest in things that would normally give you pleasure
    - Having a feeling of being down or depressed most of the time
    - Having trouble falling asleep or staying asleep
    - Having no energy and being tired most of the time
    - Having a change in appetite, usually a decrease in appetite, although some people react to stress by eating more
    - Feeling like a failure or having feelings of guilt for no good reason
    - Having trouble concentrating or thinking clearly when you need to
    - Moving slowly or being very fidgety
    - Feelings of hopelessness or even thinking about suicide

CARPE DIEM:

Check yourself for depressive symptoms. It is normal to have many of these during grief, but if you have a majority of these symptoms and they are not softening over time, talk with your doctor or counselor about it right away.

72.

SEEK HELP IF YOU HAVE DEPRESSION

- If you have had depressive symptoms for longer than two weeks, you should consult your doctor or counselor to be evaluated for possible assistance. Not everyone needs medicine, and you may just need to talk out your emotions. If you have had depression in the past or have a family history of depression, you may be more vulnerable to this biochemical problem than others in your time of grief.
- After evaluation, your physician may recommend therapy with a counselor. This "talk therapy" has been shown to improve the chemical messengers in the brain.
- Your physician may also recommend help with an antidepressant medication. These medicines may improve the level of your brain chemical messengers. Although there may be side effects from medication, especially when first starting, usually the benefit will outweigh any side effects of the medicine.
- Medication use should last at least six months to reduce the risk of recurrence of depression. Studies have shown that antidepressants can cause re-growth of cells in a part of the brain that deals with emotions, a part that may have been diminished by stress hormones. Recently it has been shown that antidepressants cause an increase in a brain-derived chemical that stimulates this re-growth.

CARPE DIEM:

If you have depression, seek help from a physician or counselor. Listen to his or her recommendations and together choose a therapy that best fits your situation.

73.

CENTER YOURSELF

- Centering yourself is about letting go of resistance and going with the movement below your feet. When you are centered, you don't let things that really don't matter in the big picture of life bother you. Therefore, it doesn't really matter what the weather is like outside, which table you are getting at a restaurant, whether the stock market goes up or down, etc. When you are centered, you are not affected by externals.
- If you are externally focused, you let little things get to you in ways they shouldn't. You get out of balance and are not centered internally. You are lost…always looking for something outside of yourself to fill you up. Yet nothing out there can.
- When you are centered, you are more aware of the environment in and around you. You have more clarity and focus, and your intuition is refined. Your fear diminishes markedly, your body becomes calm, and you know you can make it through the wilderness of grief.

CARPE DIEM:

Nurture friendships with hope-filled, centered people rather than negative or cynical people. People who are complainers are not centered and are letting the world around them affect their capacity for joy…and yours, if you allow it. When you use discernment to spend time with centered friends, you are creating a more stable environment for yourself.

74.

KEEP YOUR FRIENDS CLOSE

- Having friends and a rewarding social network has been shown to extend lifespan and improve health. Your friends will now be especially important to you as you face the sometimes overwhelming feelings of grief. How about you? Who are your close friends?

- Having a strong support network to rely on is even more important in your grieving period. During this time it is important to keep in contact with your friends and social contacts such as faith groups, clubs, and old connections.

- What is the secret to finding lasting friendships? It takes effort (but worthwhile effort). Being a good friend starts with you. People are comfortable around friends who are honest and sincere and may appreciate your openness in your time of grief. Respect your friends' boundaries and try to stay positive. Be a good listener as well as telling your story. Meet in a variety of places, like over coffee or a round of golf.

- Finding friends is easier than you might expect. Seek opportunities in your routine: talk to someone at the gym, ask a coworker to lunch, accept invitations when you can, volunteer at church or in the community, find old classmates, join a team sport, or invite neighbors over.

- Not all friends go back to childhood. The best ones are those with whom you share commonalities and can laugh together.

CARPE DIEM:

Invite a friend to lunch tomorrow. If you don't have friends living close to you, then invite a neighbor or acquaintance that you would like to befriend.

75.

REACH OUT AND TOUCH

- For many people, physical contact with another human being is healing. Touching has been recognized since ancient times as having transformative, healing powers. Touch often replaces words when words are inadequate.
- Have you hugged anyone lately? Held someone's hand? Put your arm around another human being?
- You probably know several people who enjoy hugging or physical touching. If you're comfortable with their touch, encourage it in the weeks and months to come. Touching can soothe the soul and calm the turmoil of loss in your body.
- Hug someone with whom you feel safe. Walk arm-in-arm with a neighbor.
- Getting a massage is another way of receiving healing touch. Schedule an appointment for a full-body massage today, or if this makes you uncomfortable, a shoulder and neck massage might work wonders.

CARPE DIEM:

Try hugging a close friend or family member today, even if you usually don't. You might be surprised at the comfort it brings.

76.

TAKE CARE WITH EMOTIONAL AND PHYSICAL CLOSENESS

- For some people, the thought of emotional or physical closeness with another person may be the farthest thing from their minds during their time of grief. However, grieving is a period of emotional vulnerability, and others may immediately seek the comfort of being both emotionally and physically close to someone else.
- Proceed with caution in seeking immediate emotional and physical relations, for you may need to allow yourself time to experience and work through the complex emotions of your grief before involvement with another.
- Seek support from family, trusted friends, and your social support network. If you are struggling emotionally, then talking with a physician or counselor to help work through the complexities of your grieving would be a good idea.

CARPE DIEM:

Do you think you might be seeking solace in inappropriate physical or emotional relationships right now? If so, make an appointment with a counselor to discuss this issue.

77.

ACCEPT SIMPLE GIFTS

- In your time of need, many people around you may want to help you and offer their services for basic tasks, such as cooking a meal, running errands, or cleaning your house. Some people rally around those who have suffered loss.
- At first, pride or just not wanting to put others out may prevent you from accepting these gifts. But you may not have the energy to do these simple but important tasks yourself. In your time of special needs, you must allow others to help care for you. Just like a patient in a hospital, you need to accept this intensive care from others until you gather the strength to move forward in your life.
- Those who care about you—friends, family, members of your faith community, and coworkers—would love to help you in your hour of need and can help provide some of the basics of survival, including food and the energy to do tasks around your home. Accept these gifts and allow your community to support you. This will allow you to focus on your own physical, emotional, and spiritual needs as you work through your grief.

CARPE DIEM:

If you are offered simple gifts from those you love, accept them with the love with which they are given.

78.

SPEND TIME ALONE

- Reaching out to others while you're in mourning is necessary. Mourning is hard work, and you can't get through it by yourself. But your body, by its inward turning, may signal to you that you need to withdraw and turn into yourself before reaching out to others.
- You will need alone time as you work on your needs of mourning. To slow down and turn inward, you must sometimes insist on solitude.
- Schedule alone time into each week. Go for a walk in the woods. Lock your bedroom door and read a book. Work in your garden.
- Don't shut your friends and family out altogether, but do heed the call for contemplative silence.

CARPE DIEM:

Schedule one hour of alone time into your day today.

79.

SIT IN THE SANCTUARY OF STILLNESS

- Sitting in stillness with your grief will help you honor the deeper voices of quiet wisdom that come forth from within you. As Rainer Maria Rilke observed, "Everything is gestation and then bringing forth." In honoring your need to be still, you rest for the journey.
- Personal times of stillness are a spiritual necessity. A lack of stillness hastens confusion and disorientation and results in a waning of the energy of your mind, body, and spirit. Stillness restores your life force. Grief is only transformed when you honor the quiet forces of stillness.
- Integration of grief is born out of stillness, not frantic movement forward. When you halt any instinct to attempt to "manage" your grief, other impulses such as grace, wisdom, love, and truth come forth. Any frantic attempts to quickly "move forward" or "let go" become counterproductive and deplete an already overwhelmed mind, body, and spirit. It is through sitting with stillness that your soul is ever so slowly restored.

CARPE DIEM:

Take time right now to simply sit in stillness. As you do so, you will come to recognize that "the rhythm of stillness is the teacher of contentment and peace."

80.

TAKE TIME TO BE

- In today's busy world, we do not take time for relaxation or have quiet time that allows our physiology to calm us. While you are grieving, you may be tempted to fill your days with activity to avoid your feelings of loss. This will only prolong the grief process.
- To quiet our brain activity, we need to take the time to quiet our minds without the constant intrusion of television, the internet, and mindless computer games, which often fill our quiet times with numbing activity without allowing us to engage in true relaxation.
- Taking time for a glass of iced tea on the back porch was something our rural ancestors understood, and being outdoors in nature made it easier to engage this natural relaxation response.
- Our modern society is filled with "doing," with little time for "being." To get off the treadmill of constant doing, we must take the time to do nothing in order to find our sense of being.

CARPE DIEM:

Take time for 15 minutes of doing nothing today. Set time aside each day for nothing-doing.

81.

TAKE SOME TIME OFF WORK

- Typically, our society grants us three days "bereavement leave" and then expects us to return to work as if nothing happened. Your body may make it clear to you that you can't possibly function at work this quickly and you may struggle for weeks and months after the death.
- Even if the death was long ago, you may want to take some time off work to complete a project, to travel, or to reassess your life.
- Some companies will grant extended leaves of absence or sabbaticals in some situations.
- If you simply can't take off additional time, request that your workload be lightened for the next several months. Ask to work a four-day week.

CARPE DIEM:

Take a spiritual day off today. Spend the day resting or doing something restorative.

82.

SCHEDULE SOMETHING THAT GIVES YOU PLEASURE EACH DAY

- Often grieving people struggle with getting up in the morning. When they awaken, even if they have had a peaceful night's sleep, they're confronted with the brutal reality that their loved one is gone forever.
- It's hard to look forward to each day when you know you will be experiencing pain and sadness. To counterbalance your normal and necessary mourning, give yourself a reason to get out of bed in the morning. Your body needs pleasant experiences to feel well.
- Reading, baking, going for a walk, having lunch with a friend, playing computer games—do whatever brings you enjoyment.
- On the flip side, many grieving people also feel guilty about having fun or experiencing pleasure. *I must be an awful person if I can have fun when the one I care about is dead, they think. If I have fun, that must mean I didn't totally love the person I lost.* Or: *My loved one is dead and has been deprived of the pleasures of life. What right do I have to experience pleasure?*
- Over time you'll come to realize that seeking happiness does not diminish your love for the person who died; the two can and should coexist. Like many grieving people, you may also grow to believe that you owe it to your loved one to make the most of each and every day.

CARPE DIEM:

What's on tap for today? Plan on doing something you enjoy, no matter how hectic your schedule.

83.

LAUGH

- Humor is one of the most healing gifts of humanity. Laughter restores hope and assists us in surviving the pain of grief. It helps us feel peace in both mind and body.
- Don't fall into the trap of thinking that laughing means you don't miss the person who died. Laughing doesn't mean you are not in mourning.
- Sometimes it helps to think about what the person who died would want for you. Wouldn't she want you to laugh and continue to find joy in life, even in the midst of your sorrow?
- You can only embrace the pain of your loss a little at a time, in doses. In between the doses, it's perfectly normal, even necessary, to love and laugh.
- Remember the fun times you shared with the person who died. Remember his sense of humor. Remember his grin and the sound of his laughter.
- It has been said that laughter is a form of internal jogging. Not only is it enjoyable, it is good for you. Studies show that smiling, laughing, and feeling good enhance your immune system and make you healthier. If you act happy, you may even begin to feel some happiness in your life again.

CARPE DIEM:

Close your eyes right now and try to remember the smile and laughter of the person who died.

84.

BE A KID AGAIN

- Sometimes we all just need to go back to a time when we were innocent and carefree, before loss touched our lives. Our bodies and minds were free from the strain of grieving.
- You can do it. How long has it been since you went wading in a stream or running through the sprinkler? How about jumping into a pile of leaves? Or shuffling barefoot across freshly mown grass? When's the last time you built a sandcastle?
- It is the nature of children to live for the moment and appreciate today. All of us would benefit from a little more childlike wonder.
- Do something childish—blow bubbles, skip rope, visit a toy store, fly a kite, climb a tree.
- If kids aren't already in your life, make arrangements to spend some time with them. Volunteer at a local school. Take a friend's children to the park one afternoon.

CARPE DIEM:

Right now, leave your inhibitions behind. Go do one of your favorite childhood activities. You deserve this "time-out" from your overwhelming grief.

85.

LISTEN TO THE MUSIC

- Music can be very healing to mourners because it helps us access our feelings, both happy and sad. Music can soothe the tension in your body, nurture your heart, and renew your spirit.
- All types of music can be healing—rock and roll, classical, blues, folk.
- Consider listening to music you normally don't, perhaps the opera or the symphony. Or make a recording of your favorite songs, all together on one CD or iPod playlist.
- Do you play an instrument or sing? Allow yourself the time to try these activities again soon.
- What kind of music did the one you've lost love? Get out their old CDs and spend a rainy afternoon listening to the music.
- Because music is the language of the soul, it can also be painful at times. If music brings comfort, then listen. If not, don't.

CARPE DIEM:

Visit a music store today and sample a few tracks. Or go online and sample some iTunes or MP3 files. Buy yourself the music that moves you the most.

86.

FIND COMFORT IN THE ELEMENTS

- Ancient scientists thought the world was made up of the four elements of air, earth, fire, and water. By definition, elements are pure, basic, simple. If you try you can find comfort and meaning in each of them. In some way each offer sustenance for our bodies and souls.
- Air: Breathe deeply. Practice yogic breathing. Stand in the wind.
- Fire: Light a candle in your love one's memory. Build a fire in a fireplace and sit in spiritual contemplation while you watch the flames dance. Feel the warmth on your skin.
- Earth: Garden. Plant bulbs. Start a compost pile. Feel connected to the earth.
- Water: Take a long bath. Go for a swim. Walk in the rain. Play in the sprinkler.

CARPE DIEM:

Each of the twelve signs of the zodiac is associated with one of the four elements. Look up which element your zodiac sign represents, what the element means astrologically speaking, and contemplate whether you think it's a true fit for you.

87.

GO TO THE WATER

- Many people find water to have a natural, healing quality during times of grief and loss. The gentle feeling of ocean waves washing up on the shoreline, the trickling of a mountain stream, the serenity of a quiet pond—all of these aquatic sensations can offer comfort.
- Water invites you to return to the womb – to experience the sounds you heard before being born. Water soothes the body and the soul. When you spend time near water, you connect back to its soothing natural flow, allowing it to caress your wounded heart and return you back home refreshed.
- Experiencing the tranquility that water brings into your life, you seek to match its serenity, and in doing so, you become calm in mind and body. Water reaches out to you in ways that calm your nerves and connect you with what is natural.
- Seek out opportunities to be near water and breathe in the beauty and wonder of nature. Close your eyes and repeat the following affirmation: "Water is pure and precious; water is healing; water is life."

CARPE DIEM:

Schedule one hour of time to spend near the water sometime within the next three days. Be quiet and listen as the water soothes your body and renews your soul.

88.

USE SPIRITUALITY TO CONNECT MIND, BODY, AND SPIRIT

- Many researchers feel there is a strong connection between the mind, the spirit, and the body. In your time of grieving, you may need to tend to your spiritual needs, which may in turn help your mental and physical health.
- With the death of a loved one, you can become imbalanced in mind, body, and spirit as you deal with the pain of your loss. You may have symptoms both physical and psychological, and you may even develop a sense of spiritual crisis. However, by attending to your spiritual needs regularly, you can work your way through this imbalance.
- By seeking spiritual fulfillment through prayer, meditation, or religious services, you can also improve mind and body. Since they are connected, if you improve one of these realms, the others will also improve, bringing more balance in your life.

CARPE DIEM:

Commit to doing a spiritual practice once each day this week (prayer, meditation, walking a labyrinth, whatever feels right), and at the end of the week, see if you feel better in mind, body, and spirit.

89.

IMPROVE YOUR HEALTH THROUGH SPIRITUALITY

- During your grieving process, you may find the need to get in touch with your religious or spiritual beliefs. In fact, this quest may help you find meaning and purpose as you move forward in your life. Not only can it help you cope with your loss, but spirituality has been shown to be a healthy activity.
- People who attend religious services regularly tend to be healthier, and studies show they have a lower risk of death than those who do not attend.
- Prayer and meditation seem to be associated with improved immune system function and fewer episodes of chronic inflammation.
- The benefits extend to mental health as well, and people who identify themselves as religious and practice prayer and meditation have lower rates of depression.
- Science tells us that religious people take better care of themselves, are more socially integrated, and have a better support system to help them cope with stressful life events like the death of a loved one.

CARPE DIEM:

Purposefully combine spirituality with exercise by walking to services at a nearby place of worship today.

90.

PRAY

- Prayer is mourning because prayer means taking your feelings and articulating them to someone else. Even when you pray silently, you're forming words for your thoughts and feelings, and you're offering up those words to a presence outside yourself.
- Someone wise once noted, "Our faith is capable of reaching the realm of mystery."
- Did you know that real medical studies have shown that prayer can actually help people heal? Prayer can help heal mind, body, and soul.
- If you believe in a higher power, pray. Pray for the person who died. Pray for your questions about life and death to be answered. Pray for the strength to embrace your pain and to go on to find continued meaning in life and living. Pray for others affected by this death.
- Many places of worship have prayer lists. Call yours and ask that your name be added to the prayer list. On worship days, the whole congregation will pray for you. Often many individuals will pray at home for those on the prayer list, as well.

CARPE DIEM:

Bow your head right now and say a silent prayer. If you are out of practice, don't worry. Just let your thoughts flow naturally.

91.

SPEND TIME IN "THIN" PLACES

- In the Celtic tradition, "thin places" are spots where the separation between the physical world and the spiritual world seems tenuous. Truly, they are places where the veil between Heaven and earth, between the holy and the everyday, are so thin that when we are near them, we intuitively sense the timeless, boundless spiritual.
- There is a Celtic saying that Heaven and earth are only three feet apart, but in thin places that distance is even smaller.
- Thin places are usually outdoors, often where water and land meet or land and sky come together. You might find thin places on a riverbank, a beach, or a mountaintop. You often need physical exertion to get there, which is good for your body, and the peace you find in these areas can calm your mind and soothe your spirit.
- Go to thin places to pray, to walk, or simply to sit in the presence of the holy.

CARPE DIEM:

Your thin places are anywhere that fills you with awe and a sense of wonder. They are spots that refresh your spirits and make you feel closer to God. Go to at thin place today and sit in contemplative silence.

92.

OBSERVE THE SABBATH

- The word "Sabbath" comes from the old Hebrew *shabbath*, which means literally "to rest."
- Just as God rested on the seventh day of creation, Jews and Christians "keep the Sabbath" by resting and connecting with God on Saturday or Sunday, respectively.
- Those who strictly keep the Sabbath do not work whatsoever on their day of rest. Just as God rested, during grief your body is telling you it needs a day of rest.
- You may choose to strictly observe a religious Sabbath as a day of renewal and connection with your Maker. Or you may choose to rest and rejuvenate one other day of the week as a way to embrace your spirituality. It will be a day of rest and rejuvenation for your grief-stricken body as well.
- If you observe a Sabbath day, you will be dedicating a portion of your life to your spiritual well-being. And that, regardless of your doctrine or creed, is a healthy, healing, ennobling practice.

CARPE DIEM:

Observe the Sabbath this week. Create Sabbath-day rituals that safeguard this day as a sacrosanct spiritual day.

93.

DON'T BE ALARMED BY "GRIEFBURSTS"

- Sometimes heightened periods of sadness overwhelm grieving people. These times can seem to come out of nowhere and can be frightening and painful.
- Even long after the death, something as simple as a sound, a smell, or a phrase can bring on a "griefburst." You might hear a name, see an object, or touch a fabric that suddenly reminds you of the one you have lost. This may well be a part of the physiology of our bodies reacting to a loss before we even realize it.
- Allow yourself to experience griefbursts without shame or self-judgment, no matter where and when they occur. (Sooner or later, one will probably happen when you are surrounded by people, maybe even strangers.) If you would feel more comfortable, retreat somewhere private when these strong feelings surface.
- Don't isolate yourself in an attempt to protect yourself from griefbursts. Staying cooped up at home all the time is not self-compassion, it is self-destruction.

CARPE DIEM:

Create an action plan for your next griefburst. For example, you might plan to drop whatever you are doing and go for a walk or record your thoughts in a journal.

94.

UNDERSTAND YOU ARE NOT CRAZY

- It is not unusual for people who have lost someone close to them to clearly see or hear the person about the house, and sometimes even have a conversation. These vivid visual and auditory experiences seem miraculous (and maybe they are). But they are a normal part of grief.

- Sometimes intense grief reactions can be mistaken by caregivers as severe psychiatric illness, and you may even feel "crazy" for having experienced them. Having these episodes does not mean you are "losing it" or need to be on medication. They are simply symptoms of your intense emotional state.

- Your emotions may be so overwhelming that you may have trouble focusing and dealing with the everyday complexities of life. Conversely, some people experience emotional numbing and distancing from those around them, even those who care.

- If you experience some or all of these things, rest assured that you are not "sick" or "crazy." But you may need some time and nurturing before you work your way through these strong emotions.

CARPE DIEM:

The next time you feel crazy in your time of grief, or you experience crazy physical symptoms, talk to someone you know to be a good listener about them.

95.

BE PATIENT

- You've probably realized by now that healing in grief does not usually happen quickly. And because your grief is never truly "over," you are on a lifelong journey.
- In our hurry-up North American culture, patience can be especially hard to come by. We have all been conditioned to believe that if we want something, we should be able to get it instantly.
- Yet your grief will not heed anyone's timetable—even your own. Be patient with yourself. Be patient with those around you. You are doing the best you can, as are they.
- Practicing patience means relinquishing control. Just as you cannot truly control your life, you cannot control your grief. Yes, you can set your intentions to embrace your grief and take steps to mourn well, and these practices will certainly serve you well on your journey, but you cannot control the particulars of what life will continue to lay before you.

CARPE DIEM:

When you are feeling impatient, silently repeat this phrase: "*Let nothing disturb thee; Let nothing dismay thee; All things pass; God never changes. Patience attains all that it strives for. He who has God finds he lacks nothing: God alone suffices.*" – Saint Teresa of Avila

96.

RECOGNIZE THE DUAL ASPECT OF CHANGE

- Loss can be overwhelming, and it may be difficult to move forward in any positive manner. However, it is important to remember the Chinese symbol for change is a combination of the symbols for crisis and opportunity. As you move from your survival mode of grief, you may be able to see the opportunity for you to move forward with your life and maybe even improve your health.
- Thus change has a dual identity. Even with the searing pain of loss, it is important to recognize that there is opportunity to look at where your life goes from here. Change not only brings a feeling of crisis, it also creates opportunities for you to look at the basis of your life, why you are here, and what you want to do with the rest of your life. We often do not take the time to consider these important questions. Now may be your opportunity.
- Take the opportunity to look at your life and write down what you consider important. (Was taking care of your body on the list?) Then write down how much of your time you spend doing these important things. If you are not spending much time on what you believe is essential, it is important for you to take the opportunity to change.

CARPE DIEM:

Make a point each day to be sure you are doing the things that are truly important to you.

97.

FIND WHAT GIVES MEANING TO YOUR LIFE

- You may start to examine your own life as you contemplate the passing of the life of the person you love. It may bring you to the realization of your own mortality.
- None of us will live forever, but we often live life in a bit of a daze and spend our time doing things we feel we *must* do, rather than taking the time to prioritize what we really *want* to do, deep down.
- You've heard the saying "that which does not kill me makes me stronger." In other words, when you are challenged in your life by overwhelming events, like the death of someone close, you must find the strength to persevere, and this process of digging deep within yourself can make you a stronger human being. But to make this spiritual leap, you need to take the time to care for your own being.
- Use the opportunity of the stress of your loss to examine your own life and to explore exactly what it is that makes your life worthwhile. Think about what you would like to do with the rest of your life. Find what will make your life worthwhile and fill your life with meaning.

CARPE DIEM:

Take a sheet of paper and list the most important things that give meaning to your life. Now write down how you will spend more time on meaningful activities.

98.

FEEL GOOD ABOUT YOURSELF

- Studies point to the importance of positive thinking for sound mental health. A positive attitude has also been linked to the physical side of health. It may boost immunity, aid recovery, and help us overcome other ailments. A positive attitude can also help you get through the mental and physical stressors of the grief process.

- Still, viewing life on the bright side does not come naturally to everyone. It could take some intentional changes in how you view life and your own identity and self image.

- Start by studying your positive features. What are your strengths and what do you enjoy? What would make you satisfied in life? Who are your favorite people, and what makes you laugh? When was the last time you had a good laugh out loud? What are your greatest accomplishments, and what do you have to look forward to in the future?

- We all have weakness and traits we would like to change. We all at some time wish we were smarter or more successful. It's important to stay focused on your merits and nurture a healthy self-esteem and not be pulled down by your perceived faults. Never lose sight of your goodness and unique qualities. This knowledge will help you grow and succeed, even in adverse times of grief. Hold your head up, smile, and be proud of who you are. This will not only help your state of mind, but it will improve your health as well.

CARPE DIEM:

Make a list of your positive traits today. Take time to allow yourself to feel good about these traits.

99.

CHOOSE TO LIVE

- Death often leaves mourners feeling powerless. You were powerless to prevent the death, and you're powerless to reverse it. But you can regain a feeling of power by deciding to take control of the rest of your life.
- Will you merely exist for the remainder of your days, or will you choose to truly live?
- Many mourners take up a new life direction after a sudden death. Has the death given you new perspective on life? How can you choose to act on this new perspective? Will you take better care of yourself in both body and mind?
- What did the person who died love in life? How can you help nurture the love in the world in an ongoing, positive way?
- Sometimes choosing to live simply means living mindfully, with an appreciation for all that is good and beautiful and with a deep, abiding kindness to others. It may mean taking care of yourself and others by choosing healthy ways to care for your minds and bodies.
- As a wise person once observed, "When old words die out on the tongue, new melodies spring from the heart."

CARPE DIEM:

Do one small thing today that demonstrates your desire to live rather than merely existing.

100.

BELIEVE IN YOUR CAPACITY TO HEAL

- Veteran grievers would want us to give you one simple message: You will survive.
- If your loss is recent, you may think you cannot get through this. You can and you will. It may be excruciatingly difficult, yes, and you must take the steps to take care of your body while you heal. But over time and with the love and support of others, your grief will soften and you will find ways to be happy again. There will come a day when the death is not the first thing you think of when you wake up in the morning.
- Many mourners also struggle with feeling they don't *want* to survive. Again, those who have gone before you want you to know that while this feeling is normal, it will pass. One day in the not-too-distant future, you will feel that life is worth living again. For now, think of how important you are to your children, your partner, your parents, your siblings, and your friends.
- As you actively mourn, you may also choose not to simply survive, but to truly live. The remainder of your life can be full and rich and satisfying if you choose life over mere existence.

CARPE DIEM:

Create a vision board for your future. Grab a stack of old magazines and newspapers and cut out images that represent your hopes and dreams. Include a photo of the person who died on your vision board, since remembering the past and continuing to love this person will also be part of your future. Hang this vision board where you will see it often.

A FINAL WORD

In the beginning of this book, we acknowledged that to be "bereaved" means "to be torn apart" and to have "special needs." One of your most important needs is to take care of your physical self. As we have noted throughout this resource, caring for your physical self will put your body in a more balanced state, and a body that is more balanced is in a better position to heal itself.

Physical self-care fortifies you for the ongoing ebbs and flows of your grief journey, a journey that leaves you profoundly affected and deeply changed. Your commitment to care for yourself physically is an integral part of your ultimate healing. Then and only then do you go on to find meaning in your continued living.

Once you have the courage and fortitude to care for your physical self and do your work of mourning, your open and grateful heart will fill your soul with love and light!

We also believe that when you care for yourself physically, you create an appreciation for living each remaining moment of your life, for finding hidden treasures everywhere—a child's smile, a beautiful sunrise, a flower in bloom, a friend's gentle touch.

Yes, taking good care of yourself allows you to be open to the mystery and live fully in the present while, at the same time, remembering your past and embracing your future.

Grief instinctively invites our bodies to slow down, turn inward, and take care of ourselves. Walt Whitman wrote, "I celebrate myself." In taking good care of your physical self, you are celebrating that you have the opportunity to be alive and live on this earth. To come to recognize the preciousness of life is a superb opportunity for celebration!

Grief instinctively invites you to simplify your life and to be open to giving and receiving love. You need and deserve a sense of belonging, a sense of meaning, a sense of purpose! In caring for your physical self, you plant the seeds that allow these important needs to bloom in your life. We truly hope this little book has served and will continue to serve as a gentle companion.

Bless you. We wish you peace and a healthy life!

THE MOURNER'S CODE

Ten Self-Compassionate Principles

Though you should reach out to others as you journey through grief, you should not feel obligated to accept the unhelpful responses you may receive from some people. You are the one who is grieving, and as such, you have certain "rights" no one should try to take away from you.

The following list is intended both to empower you to heal and to decide how others can and cannot help. This is not to discourage you from reaching out to others for help, but rather to assist you in distinguishing useful responses from hurtful ones.

1. **You have the right to experience your own unique grief.** No one else will grieve in exactly the same way you do. So, when you turn to others for help, don't allow them to tell you what you should or should not be feeling.
2. **You have the right to talk about your grief.** Talking about your grief will help you heal. Seek out others who will allow you to talk as much as you want, as often as you want, about your grief. If at times you don't feel like talking, you also have the right to be silent.
3. **You have the right to feel a multitude of emotions.** Confusion, numbness, disorientation, fear, guilt and relief are just a few of the emotions you might feel as part of your grief journey. Others may try to tell you that feeling angry, for example, is wrong. Don't take these judgmental responses to heart. Instead, find listeners who will accept your feelings without condition.
4. **You have the right to be tolerant of your physical and emotional limits.** Your feelings of loss and sadness will probably leave you feeling fatigued. Respect what your body and mind are telling you. Get daily rest. Eat balanced meals.

And don't allow others to push you into doing things you don't feel ready to do.

5. **You have the right to experience "griefbursts."** Sometimes, out of nowhere, a powerful surge of grief may overcome you. This can be frightening, but it is normal and natural. Find someone who understands and will let you talk it out.

6. **You have the right to make use of ritual.** The funeral ritual does more than acknowledge the death of someone loved. It helps provide you with the support of caring people. More importantly, the funeral is a way for you to mourn. If others tell you the funeral or other healing rituals such as these are silly or unnecessary, don't listen.

7. **You have the right to embrace your spirituality.** If faith is a part of your life, express it in ways that seem appropriate to you. Allow yourself to be around people who understand and support your religious beliefs. If you feel angry at God, find someone to talk with who won't be critical of your feelings of hurt and abandonment.

8. **You have the right to search for meaning.** You may find yourself asking, "Why did he or she die? Why this way? Why now?" Some of your questions may have answers, but some may not. And watch out for the clichéd responses some people may give you. Comments like, "It was God's will" or "Think of what you have to be thankful for" are not helpful and you do not have to accept them.

9. **You have the right to treasure your memories.** Memories are one of the best legacies that exist after the death of someone loved. You will always remember. Instead of ignoring your memories, find others with whom you can share them.

10. **You have the right to move toward your grief and heal.** Reconciling your grief will not happen quickly. Remember, grief is a process, not an event. Be patient and tolerant with yourself and avoid people who are impatient and intolerant with you. Neither you nor those around you must forget that the death of someone loved changes your life forever.

WANTED: YOUR PHYSICAL SELF-CARE IDEAS

Please help us write the next edition of this book. We will plan to update and rewrite this book every few years. For this reason we would really like to hear from you. Please write and let us know about your experience with this book.

If an Idea is particularly helpful to you, let us know. Better yet, send us an Idea you have that you think other fellow mourners might find helpful. When you write to us, you are "helping us help others" and inspiring us to be more effective grief companions, authors, and educators.

Thank you for your help. Please write to us at:

Center for Loss and Life Transition
3735 Broken Bow Road
Fort Collins, CO 80526
Or email us at DrWolfelt@centerforloss.com or go to this website, www.centerforloss.com.

My idea:

____

____

____

____

____

My name and mailing address:

____

____

____

ALSO BY ALAN WOLFELT

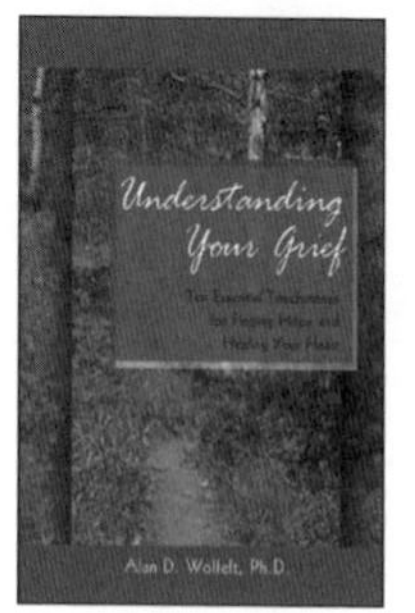

Understanding Your Grief

Ten Essential Touchstones for Finding Hope and Healing Your Heart

One of North America's leading grief educators, Dr. Alan Wolfelt has written many books about healing in grief. This book is his most comprehensive, covering the essential lessons that mourners have taught him in his three decades of working with the bereaved.

In compassionate, down-to-earth language, *Understanding Your Grief* describes ten touchstones—or trail markers—that are essential physical, emotional, cognitive, social, and spiritual signs for mourners to look for on their journey through grief.

The Ten Essential Touchstones:

1. Open to the presence of your loss.
2. Dispel misconceptions about grief.
3. Embrace the uniqueness of your grief.
4. Explore what you might experience.
5. Recognize you are not crazy.
6. Understand the six needs of mourning.
7. Nurture yourself.
8. Reach out for help.
9. Seek reconciliation, not resolution.
10. Appreciate your transformation.

Think of your grief as a wilderness—a vast, inhospitable forest. You must journey through this wilderness. To find your way out, you must become acquainted with its terrain and learn to follow the sometimes hard-to-find trail that leads to healing. In the wilderness of your grief, the touchstones are your trail markers. They are the signs that let you know you are on the right path. When you learn to identify and rely on the touchstones, you will find your way to hope and healing.

ISBN 978-1-879651-35-7 • 176 pages • softcover • $14.95

All Dr. Wolfelt's publications can be ordered by mail from:
Companion Press
3735 Broken Bow Road
Fort Collins, CO 80526
(970) 226-6050
www.centerforloss.com

ALSO BY ALAN WOLFELT

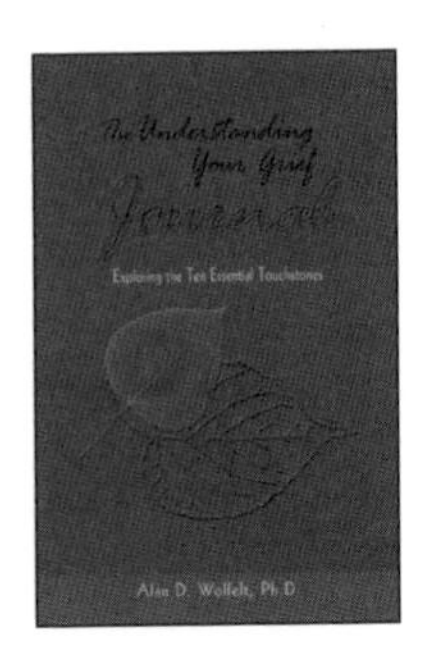

The Understanding Your Grief Journal

Exploring the Ten Essential Touchstones

Writing can be a very effective form of mourning, or expressing your grief outside yourself. And it is through mourning that you heal in grief.

The Understanding Your Grief Journal is a companion workbook to Dr. Wolfelt's *Understanding Your Grief*. Designed to help mourners explore the many facets of their unique grief through journaling, this compassionate book interfaces with the ten essential touchstones. Throughout, journalers are asked specific questions about their own unique grief journeys as they relate to the touchstones and are provided with writing space for the many questions asked.

Purchased as a set together with *Understanding Your Grief*, this journal is a wonderful mourning tool and safe place for those in grief. It also makes an ideal grief support group workbook.

ISBN 978-1-879651-39-5 • 150 pages • softcover • $14.95

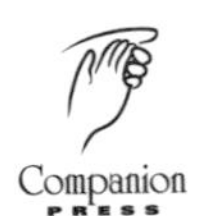

All Dr. Wolfelt's publications can be ordered by mail from:
Companion Press
3735 Broken Bow Road
Fort Collins, CO 80526
(970) 226-6050
www.centerforloss.com

ALSO BY ALAN WOLFELT

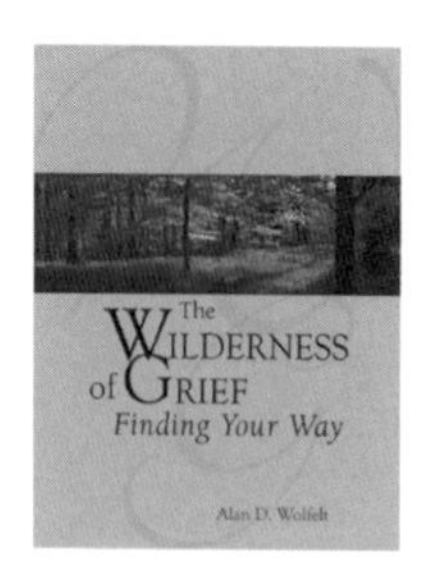

The Wilderness of Grief

Finding Your Way

A beautiful, hardcover gift book version of *Understanding Your Grief*

Understanding Your Grief provides a comprehensive exploration of grief and the ten essential touchstones for finding hope and healing your heart. *The Wilderness of Grief* is an excerpted version of *Understanding Your Grief*, making it approachable and appropriate for all mourners.

This concise book makes an excellent gift for anyone in mourning. On the book's inside front cover is room for writing an inscription to your grieving friend.

While some readers will appreciate the more in-depth *Understanding Your Grief*, others may feel overwhelmed by the amount of information it contains. For these readers we recommend *The Wilderness of Grief*. (Fans of *Understanding Your Grief* will also want a copy of *The Wilderness of Grief* to turn to in spare moments.)

The Wilderness of Grief is an ideal book for the bedside or coffee table. Pick it up before bed and read just a few pages. You'll be carried off to sleep by its gentle, affirming messages of hope and healing.

ISBN 978-1-879651-52-4 • 128 pages • hardcover • $15.95

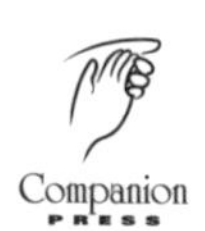

All Dr. Wolfelt's publications can be ordered by mail from:
Companion Press
3735 Broken Bow Road
Fort Collins, CO 80526
(970) 226-6050
www.centerforloss.com

ALSO BY ALAN WOLFELT

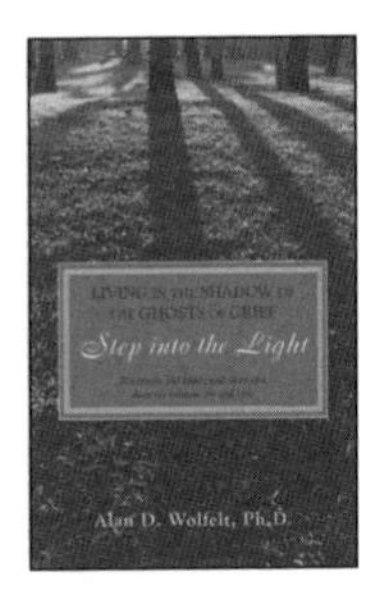

Living in the Shadow of the Ghosts of Grief

Step into the Light

Reconcile old losses and open the door to infinite joy and love

"*Accumulated, unreconciled loss affects every aspect of our lives.* Living in the Shadow *is a beautifully written compass with the needle ever-pointing in the direction of hope.*"
— Greg Yoder, grief counselor

"*So often we try to dance around our grief. This book offers the reader a safe place to do the healing work of "catch-up" mourning, opening the door to a life of freedom, authenticity and purpose.*"
— Kim Farris-Luke, bereavement coordinator

Are you depressed? Anxious? Angry? Do you have trouble with trust and intimacy? Do you feel a lack of meaning and purpose in your life? You may well be living in the shadow of the ghosts of grief.

When you suffer a loss of any kind—whether through abuse, divorce, job loss, the death of someone loved or other transitions, you naturally grieve inside. To heal your grief, you must express it. That is, you must mourn your grief. If you don't, you will carry your grief into your future, and it will undermine your happiness for the rest of your life.

This compassionate guide will help you learn to identify and mourn your carried grief so you can go on to live the joyful, whole life you deserve.

ISBN 978-1-879651-51-7 • 160 pages • softcover • $13.95

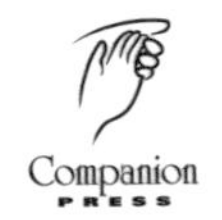

All Dr. Wolfelt's publications can be ordered by mail from:
Companion Press
3735 Broken Bow Road
Fort Collins, CO 80526
(970) 226-6050
www.centerforloss.com

ALSO BY ALAN WOLFELT

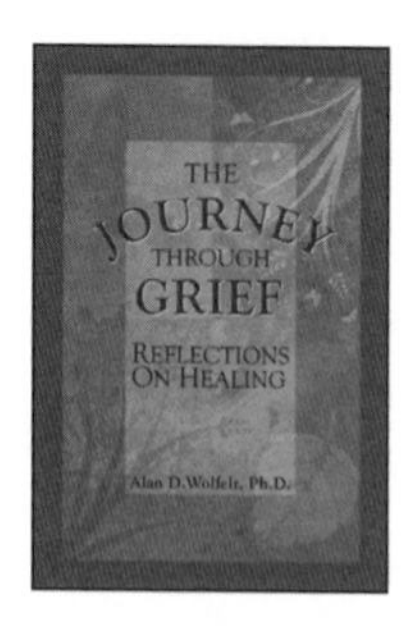

The Journey Through Grief

Reflections On Healing
Second Edition

This popular hardcover book makes a wonderful gift for those who grieve, helping them gently engage in the work of mourning. Comforting and nurturing, *The Journey Through Grief* doses mourners with the six needs of mourning, helping them soothe themselves at the same time it helps them heal.

Back by popular demand, we are now offering *The Journey Through Grief* again in hardcover. The hardcover version of this beautiful book makes a wonderful, healing gift for the newly bereaved.

This revised, second edition of *The Journey Through Grief* takes Dr. Wolfelt's popular book of reflections and adds space for guided journaling, asking readers thoughtful questions about their unique mourning needs and providing room to write responses.

The Journey Through Grief is organized around the six needs that all mourners must yield to—indeed embrace—if they are to go on to find continued meaning in life and living. Following a short explanation of each mourning need is a series of brief, spiritual passages that, when read slowly and reflectively, help mourners work through their unique thoughts and feelings. *The Journey Through Grief* is being used by many faith communities as part of their grief support programs.

ISBN 978-1-879651-11-1 • hardcover • 176 pages • $21.95

All Dr. Wolfelt's publications can be ordered by mail from:
Companion Press
3735 Broken Bow Road
Fort Collins, CO 80526
(970) 226-6050
www.centerforloss.com